For Sophia, my forever girl.

Lean in, I have something to tell you.

Dear woman in deep sleep,

It's time to wake up to your life. You know there is something miss-ing, deep down. As that space that once knew peace and content-ment fills with resentment, with fatigue and hopelessness, it seems too hard to even begin to unpack the hurt. You've tried so many things and ended up numbing out with modern convenience. Your deepest desires are a whisper invading your senses, letting you know they want out, they want to be seen, to be felt, to be lived. Don't ignore them any longer. Honor your true desires. Own your sensu-ality. Liberate your divine feminine. Yes, it is time to Return to Her. Hold my hand. I'll help you find her.

Lesley

INTRODUCTION

UNBECOMING WHO YOU are is necessary to becoming who you are meant to be; the bright, joyful woman inside you under protective custody, just waiting for permission to emerge. Your authentic self - unfiltered, unvarnished - is exquisite. Your journey to unbecoming has a guarantee: it will involve falls, heartbreak, grief, immense bravery and the most courage you have ever summoned in your life. This is guaranteed. This guarantee also includes joy, courage, happiness, bliss and liberation like you have never known. All wrapped up in a blanket of comforting freedom, luscious pleasure and ease.

It's that easy, yes. But it sounds absolutely daunting. What will become of all of the people you have taken care of before your unbecoming? They will still be there. Those who have the capacity to care for themselves will be entrusted to do so. Those who need nurturing and support to grow into who they will become will follow your lead, with gentle guidance will emerge as the people they were born to be. Your actions will become their mirror. Your courageous steps towards owning your freedom and pleasure on your terms will contribute to breaking the cycle of martyrdom and compassion fatigue burning out woman all over the planet and instead replace it with permission to bloom where they are planted, unapologetically.

How you do anything is how you do everything. So how you

show up at work, with family and with friends, is how you show up in bed, in love and in relationships. Do you give it everything you have or are you editing yourself so acceptance into the external validation club is guaranteed? Take the road less travelled and find yourself. Rediscover your pleasure and taste the palate of your sensuality all over again.

This book chronicles the feminine journey from blindness to light, from deafness to wisdom, from dullness to beauty. I will share my personal journey as well as the trips other sisters have taken towards wholeness. Your greatest desires are available to you right now.

Your life mirrors your beliefs. It is a reflection of your declarations of wants, needs, fears and desires. Are all these things serving you or are you operating on autopilot? Are they just old habits clogging up space? Make room for your desires to manifest themselves. Let your senses guide your creativity and fuel your dreams. Do it. You are the artist of your life. Create what is most important to you.

What I know to be true is this: who you are right now, as you turn page 1 of this book, as you begin an exploration of awakening, is enough. Those big lofty goals? 100 pages from now you will know that who you were when you started reading this book is enough to manifest your desires and reawaken your soulful sensual self.

Whatever your body size, shape, whatever your relationship to yourself, sensuality is the way in, sister. Acknowledge and honour your senses, your innate sensual knowing and history. Your inner desire compass. You have to be willing to feel the pain of what you've been avoiding in order to experience the pleasure you have been seeking. There is no emotional editing. Reclaim your body and reawaken your sacred feminine wisdom.

Another truth that needs to be recognized is this: you don't know yourself completely until you know your sensual self. This is where your life force operates from; where the seat of your creativity, your freedom and sense of connection lives and breathes. We as women are conditioned to keep Her small and private when all she wants to do is show Herself. And most of us will filter how she shows up.

Healing our sensual selves is about honouring our sensual flow, challenging beliefs that restrict our glow and creating a sensual experience that is truly unique to us. There is no blueprint for sexual expression. It is yours. As you reclaim your sexual power, you will become more confident and clear about who you are as a sensual woman in the world. This will extend to every other part of life. Opening up to the sensual woman within is about examining your relationship to receiving. Your true sexual nature is unique to you, no one can it take away, it can never be broken.

Your divine feminine is trying to emerge, not to steal the show, but she's desiring some of the spotlight. How does it feel to shine some light on her?

So what does a fully expressed and awakened woman look like?

You. Exactly like you. It's true.

Dear beautiful woman,

This book is your invitation to explore your sensual side uninhibited, to dive deep below the surface to really get to know your desires and create an action plan to put those desires into motion. You'll receive structured concepts about sensual flow and poetic backup from women who have walked the walk before you as well as find support in questions and worksheets designed to reveal and amplify your answers.

> *"Even the most repressed woman has a secret life, with secret thoughts and secret feelings which are lush and wild, that is natural. Even the most captured woman guards the place of the wildish self, for she knows there will be a loophole, an aperture a chance and she will hightail it and escape."*
>
> Clarissa Pinkola Estes

Ladies, this book is your direction to that portal, that loophole that lets the pleasure in. And there is no closing the portal. Once you're in, you're in. There is no going back to the way life was. You will receive some backlash and some hard feelings from others once you open up the portal to your feminine. The truth is: you cannot control what other people project but what you can control is whether or not you allow those projections to control you. When you stop looking for approval externally, you gain so much energy back. Energy that you can now use to manifest your desires, uncover pleasure and access the deep feminine parts of yourself that have been dormant for so long. So what is the catalyst to take this leap?

Sometimes we have to get so sick of our inner selves that we start looking for the portal in order to make a change. Pain, anxiety and discomfort are signs that an inner revolution is on its way. Start preparing. Expanding your comfort zone is extremely uncomfortable. You can't see the exceptional things waiting for you on the other side if you stay the same. Follow your intuition and investigate why it's guiding you towards your desires. Fall in love all over again with that part of yourself you have been ignoring for years. She needs your love, your vulnerability and your bravery.

It's time to stop playing nice out of fear of judgement and disapproval, because is it worth filling your life with people don't whole heartedly love the real you? You are soooooooo close to having everything you have ever desired.

And you have the power to make it all happen.

How? By embracing all that you are. Return to Her, and open the portal to your sensuality. Show up as the real you in the world. Create space for your inner truth to arise. Every day. Because that's what really matters on the awakening journey. And watch your desires manifest, come true and shine brighter. The portal allows you to stay open to your wild, sensual self, to open to your true nature as a woman and own your sensuality. You will come to discover, know and trust your essential sensual nature and witness what is alive and stirring within.

Your desire to wake up needs to be stronger than your desire to stay unconscious. If your desire to stay unconscious is stronger than your desire to expand, you stay stuck and asleep. The gap between your desires and your reality insidiously grows bigger every day. One day you finally pry one eye open, wipe away the sleepy dust and proclaim, "How the hell did I get here?" When you water down your essence, you lose the energy and clarity behind it.

In the moment, it is so much easier to fall back on our default settings and play small. The perception that it is safe here is false, yet it overrides our reality and conscious thinking. Returning to Her and awakening to your sensual self is all about creating new neural pathways, increasing conscious awareness of thought and beliefs and being at choice. In the moment, questioning, what is behind why I am reacting this way? What am I afraid of facing? When you consciously and repetitively choose the less travelled path, the default doesn't feel so powerful.

This is reinforced by acknowledging our choices each time we vote against the default. What is your relationship to celebrating? Does it come as an afterthought once your to do list is done? That's a fallacy. It's never done. Make celebration a priority. It is for pleasure and enjoyment. Relationship to receiving? It is all related.

It's so easy to play small. It's safe from rejection and judgement. If you showed up as yourself in all your shining delightfulness, you put yourself at risk.

Your echoes may sound something like, "If I show up as the real me, you may not like it and reject me. Therefore if I don't show you my whole self, I can't get hurt." Only it backfires and you end up creating a bigger distance and hurting yourself. You end up achieving the opposite of what it is you truly desire.

Removing the layers of sensual shame gets you one step closer to your true nature. Step out of the shadow of your sexual shame and into your sensual feminine power. Acknowledge and honour your senses and be willing to feel the pain of what you've been avoiding in order to experience the pleasure you have been seeking. There is no emotional editing when you reclaim your body and reawaken your sacred feminine wisdom.

Reclaim your original voice and make space for pleasure to roll in and fuel you. Reclaim the knowing that is at the heart of the feminine. When I gave myself permission to listen to my desires instead of minimizing them, it hit me in the place that truth needed to land. It was about becoming more of myself and releasing all that was blocking me from being who I really am and allowing my inner sensual self to emerge, on her terms.

The emergence and nurturing of Sexual Confidence is rooted in three Core Concepts:

1. ***Your primary sexual relationship is and always has been with yourself.*** You are the expert on your pleasure – no one else knows your erotic landscape better than you.

   Intimate connection with another person provides the opportunity for you to share the results of your ongoing pleasure research in ecstatic union; *to amplify and sustain vitality in your life.*

   Your partner cannot show you how to receive pleasure unless you share with them your pleasure map. It is up to you to indicate where your treasure lies so that great discoveries can be made.

2. ***Expanding your Sexual Confidence has benefits that reach far beyond the bedroom door.***

   Owning your sexual confidence is inviting. People around you are drawn in. Defining your sexual expression is far more than how you show up in bed. Sexual Confidence shows up as being emotionally *close and available* to your family, your community and in your self-assuredness at work, which can lead to greater responsibility and greater financial success. Your Sexual Confidence is a vital life force that cannot be ignored. It permeates every layer of your being. Your task is to identify how your Sexual Confidence shows up in your life, to nurture it and to utilize it. Everyone around you benefits when you make pleasure in your life a priority.

3. ***You have everything you need to experience the most sensual version of yourself today, right now.***

   It's all in you - the confidence, the language, the self-assuredness, the voice of your desires. Your pleasure is alive and well, however you may be out of practice expressing it. Your desires may be hidden and obscured behind old messages, emotional clutter and outdated expressions of fear. Your desires deserve space. You have a choice to remove the clutter and shine light into the dark corners and experience just how much pleasure your life can embody.

   A richer, fuller more sensual life is yours - if you choose it. What if you could find safety and security in your own resilience?

Achieve sensual mastery through freeing of your desires. Align your creativity with your sensuality and watch what happens. In this book, we will explore what it looks like to live a life aligned with your deepest desires. Throughout the course of this book, I will show you what awakening your sensuality looks like and challenge you along the way with questions, worksheets and exercises to stimulate your sensual side and question your motivations. You get to choose. You'll walk away with the truth inside you, illuminated so you can see your path towards greater pleasure.

The truth is this wisdom already resides inside you. She is just waiting for you to open the portal and let her play. Let's begin.

Chapter 1
Putting Sensuality in Context

Sensuality is the key to activating your power as a woman.

Consciously, I thought I was comfortable with my sensual nature but I couldn't deal with a world that constantly resisted that part of me.

Great sex is a natural byproduct of living in alignment with your truest desires.

Be who you are before all that stuff dimmed your shine. Become yourself again.

In order to start to dive below the surface of your sensuality, it is important to place it within the larger context and concept of sexuality.

> "The woman in deep sleep is one who goes about an unconscious state. She seems unaware or unfazed by the truth of her own female life the truth about women in general, the way woman in the feminine have been wounded, devalued, and limited within culture, churches, and families. She cannot see the wound or feel the pain. She has never knowledge much less confronted sexism."
>
> *Sue Monk Kidd*

BEFORE I MOVE forward and embrace sensuality, creativity and desire, I have found it helpful to place them in a context that helps explain how they relate to each other and fit into the spectrum of sexuality as a greater umbrella. Sexuality is bigger than the physical realm. It is so much more than sexual intercourse. It is how we express ourselves in the world, how we show up as male/female, being in love, feeling connected, using our power to flirt and seduce, as well as the ability to produce offspring.

The term sexuality is often interchanged with the word sex. They're both terms overheard quite often and aren't clearly defined, or even defined at all. Sexuality has no definitive definition. Why? Because each one of us defines, expresses and holds sexual agency differently, a unique expression that changes from day to day as we transition through life.

My favorite lens to examine sexuality through is the Circles of Sexuality (Figure 1), a Theoretical Model designed by Dennis Dailey, a Social Worker at the University of Missouri.

Dailey's model comprises five interlocking circles in a round pattern. I like to view them as a wheel. When each circle or topic is healthy the wheel spins freely. If not balanced, then one slice of the circle will become deflated and will always be the spoke that trips you up. Just like when you get a flat tire, you get stuck until you invest time, energy and thought into getting the momentum going again.

The five headings within Dailey's Model of Sexuality are Intimacy, Sexual Identity, Sexual Anatomy and Reproduction, Sexual Power and Sensuality.

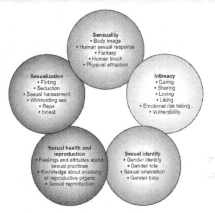

Figure 1

Intimacy

Intimacy and sensuality are close cousins. Whereas sensuality is a physical closeness, intimacy can be defined as an emotional closeness with another person. The key characteristic to intimacy is reciprocity: the ability to be emotionally close to another person and accept the same closeness in return. Intimacy includes: emotional risk taking; putting yourself out there with the risk of not being reciprocated, liking/loving another person, caring and sharing emotional vulnerability with another.

The key ingredient to intimacy is vulnerability; putting ourselves out there means the other person has the power to hurt us emotionally. Intimacy requires vulnerability, on the part of each person in the relationship. We are at our most courageous when we are willing to dive head first into genuine intimacy.

Sexual Identity

This is a concept based on binaries, encompassing three different, but related identities. The first is biological gender, our sense of being male or female, or somewhere along the binary. The second concept is gender identity, whether we identify as male or female or somewhere along the binary. This may or may not be congruent with our biological gender. The third concept is sexual orientation: who we find ourselves attracted to, the same or opposite gender or someone along the binary.

Sexual Health and Reproduction

I like to call this one, the Innies and Outies. This circle refers to all things biological and the mechanics of sexuality. It encompasses factual information about the biological processes involved in sexual intercourse, reproduction, sexually transmitted infection (STI) transmission, puberty, anatomy, contraception/STI prevention and the hormonal/nervous system cascade that occurs with orgasm. Sexy right? No. Necessary? Yes. Consider this health information and education. This is usually the beginning and the end of health education we receive in North American schools.

Sexual Power and Agency

Power and sex are intrinsically linked. The relationship shows how people behave sexually to influence, manipulation or the of control others. Sexual power shows up insidiously and blatantly every day.

It includes: flirting (using our sexual power to alert another that we are interested in emotional closeness, seduction (with mutual consent, acting on skin hunger). At this point the power can be used against us as harassment (unwanted name calling/gossiping/touching), sexual assault (nonconsensual sexual contact) and incest (nonconsensual sexual contact with a minor person within a family structure). Harassment, assault and incest are illegal and never your fault. Unresolved feelings from a historical abuse of power can interfere with optimal sexual function.

The last round out this model is the reason you're reading this book: Sensuality.

Sensuality

Sensuality is defined as an awareness and experience of feeling your body and others bodies. It is how we experience pleasure in the environment. Think of it as *{sense}-uality*; using your five senses to interact with and perceive stimuli in your environment. The stimuli enters your body through your senses - taste, smell, sight, touch and hearing. Sensuality also includes how we feel about our bodies, how we chose to experience pleasure, as well as feeling the desire to connect physically with another person, and using fantasy as a tool to increase desire and the experience that comes along with orgasm. We satiate our need for skin hunger - the need to be touched or touch another person in a loving, caring way, the need for physical closeness - with our sensuality.

Sensuality is how we experience pleasure in our environment. We return to and seek out experiences that make us feel goooood. A juicy peach, the smell of fresh cut grass, your lover's cologne, watching a woman belly dance, wet moss under your toes, the feel of freshly dried linen in the sun. All are ways I experience pleasure in my environment. Your desires and sensuality are uniquely yours. We'll dive deeper into desire in Chapter 5.

Your sensuality is the powerful keystone that supports all the roles you play in life, so you can move closer to delight, intimacy and joy and live life as a fully integrated awake person.

The concepts of sensuality and sexuality are often used interchangeably, but are not the same idea.

Teresa is a 45 year old healthcare worker and mother of three who believes that sex and sensuality are two different concepts. Her distinction between sex and sensuality is very accurate:

> The difference between sex and sensuality is subtle. When I think of sensuality, it's using all my senses. Sexuality does as well but it's more confining. Sensuality needs a wider space where sexuality is a finer tuned version of sensuality. Whenever I try to give language a feeling, I look at the opposite concept, the opposite of awakened means to be asleep, it means to be not aware, a reactionary mode, just a reflex, almost like when you hit your knee in a certain spot and it kicks out. An awakening requires more space, it's more of a time of intent and a conscious process. The more awakened I am, the more sensual depth I experience. For me, that's done through a process of inquiry and getting in touch with the now, through my senses. I slow down, I'm present in the space and it's a process.

What does sex and sensuality mean to you?

Brainstorm 20 words that you associate with sexuality. Let them spill out. List them. Place them under each heading on The Circles of Sexuality Model. Then based on honest expression and experience, give each circle a rating based on your effort. This will give you a baseline, a place to focus your future effort and energy. If your wheel spins, will it get stuck? Start your focus there and keep moving forward.

And so, with a context to place our ideas about sensuality, we can begin to dive deep and explore where your sensuality lives, what it wants to express and how to manifest those desires. Are you ready?

Take a breath and go......Give yourself permission.

CHAPTER 2
REWRITE YOUR PERMISSION SLIP

"A ship is safe in harbor, but that's not what ships are built for."

William G.T. Shedd

PERMISSION TO HAVE more pleasure being authentically you? Granted.

It's time to wake up to your life. The strange and delicious life that is yours. It may not be a smooth road, but what a story it will be. Your story. Wake up to the beauty, the luminosity and the pleasure just waiting for you to say YES and embrace it. Right here. Right now.

A part-time sensualist? That doesn't work. Meet yourself fully immersed in the beauty of what you desire. Permission to express your desires and permission to feel it are two different things. Permission and success: you cannot have one without the other.

Imagine this:

What if you gave yourself permission to listen to and hear the deepest desires tattooed on your soul? What would life be like if you chose to live in complete alignment with the dharma of your desires?

What would it look like if you didn't edit your sensuality?

I will not edit or downplay my sensual energy for fear of being labeled a slut, easy, or asking for it. My sensuality knows no shame. In the past, I have edited myself so that others could feel safe in their smallness. This does not serve either any of us. When we both play small, resentment grows and I grow to resent you for restraining my energy. And that is why I am no longer willing to edit my sensual self so that you feel safe in your smallness. I want you and your fiercely feminine self to join me unedited and free to be in touch and express our sensual selves easily and without blame. Ask yourself how you've contributed to the smallness of your sisters, your children and your friends. When you are brave and when you shine in your Shakti energy you give others around you permission to do the same.

Marianne Williamson said it best in her book, Return to Love:

Our deepest fear is not that we are inadequate. Our deepest fear is that we are powerful beyond measure. It is our light, not our darkness that most frightens us. We ask ourselves, Who am I to be brilliant, gorgeous, talented, fabulous? Actually, who are you not to be? You are a child of God. Your playing small does not serve the world. There is nothing enlightened about shrinking so that other people won't feel insecure around you. We are all meant to shine, as children do. We were born to make manifest the glory of God that is within us. It's not just in some of us; it's in everyone. And as we let our own light shine, we unconsciously give other people permission to do the same. As we are liberated from our own fear, our presence automatically liberates others."

The question is not who are you to shine and be powerful. The question is this: who are you not to shine and fully express your powerful sensual self exquisitely as you stand unedited, full of grace and full of power? Trusting we are exactly where we need to be. To ignite, expand and rise as feminine creatures. Playing small often comes from a comparison to others and a measure against their perceived successes and wins. Are your successes measured against the highlight reel of other's lives?

Is life passing you by, waiting for your how to show up, to be delivered to you?

Are you actively participating in creating the life of your dreams or sitting back, waiting for the silver platter to appear?

How are you delegating responsibility for your successes?

That is a massive amount of power to give away.

How do you feel about giving it away:

resentful?

angry?

powerless?

Feeling resentful is a complete waste of energy. Instead, imagine you are the Queen Bee.

Yes, be the Queen Bee.

Own your hive.

Create a tribe that supports your own unique fabulous vision of you.

Share what lights your fire.

Call a friend, tell your spouse, your dog, your mirror.

Say it out loud.

Do it.

I'll wait.

Did you do it? Heidi did it. Here's her story:

Heidi is a 40 year old woman, recently separated mother, who took the long road to owning her sensuality. For 29 years, she hid until she came to know and own her power.

9

I didn't grow up in house where we talked about sex. And somehow it felt like something I couldn't talk about. Other girls could, but I'd just shy away. I first had sex when I was 16 and it was pretty darn exciting. I certainly was one of those that mixed up sex and love, I felt it was an intimate connection that bound me to someone and most of the time, it wasn't. All my messages would come from movies and that's what shaped my outlook on sex. I remember my dad when I was 16, he said, "Is there ever anything that scares you?" I honestly felt like he was trying to broach the subject without saying it. And of course, all I could think of was death.

In my 20s, I was more of myself and more relaxed and was able to attract guys I liked. In my late 20s, I remember cuddling with my mom one day and bringing up the topic of sex and having the first conversation about sex, ever. I must have been 29 years old. Now I'm almost 49, and for the past 10 years, it's been easy for me to talk about sex. I have no qualms talking about sex. Between 29-39, my walls around the subject dropped and I was able to have friendships and subsequent relationships. And then I met the guy who was to be my husband. We started as friends. We had an emotional closeness before we had a physical closeness.

What woke up in me? I had 2 psychotic episodes and they were wake up calls for me. Cognitive Therapy changed my thinking. I dropped the "always" and "shoulds" and stopped the "nevers". I slowly started taking down the walls and I think it was a way for my family to stop controlling me so much. I felt like an elastic band, pulled between what they wanted and what I wanted. It was like the elastic band just snapped. At this point, that gave me space and I took back control of my life and learned how to trust me. I love being able to talk about sex, there is a lot of humour that comes with it.

Sexual expression is a direct expression of joy, to share with another person. I see a relationship between our spirituality and our creativity. The more in touch we are with our inner joy and light and passion, the more we want to express it in our unique creative ways. One becomes alive and the other thrives too. Sexuality. Creativity. Spirituality. They all affect each other.

Your sensuality is the fuel of your vitality. You have to have a powerful emotional attachment to the change you want to happen. Your why has to be bigger than your why-nots. Why is it important to you? Why is it important now? Your change has to come from a passionate motivated place. What makes you wake up every morning? Know what this is. Get clear. Wear it proudly. Choose how you want to be in the world and the greatest way to share your shining gift.

Remember: You are the gift.

What if you also surrendered to the ugly cries with their snot and sobs as part of your journey to living in complete alignment with who you are and what you desire? Does it make you nauseated? I hope so. You are moving in the right direction, the direction of your desires. Keep going it's worth it. Nausea and all. You've got this! Moving out of your comfort zone and giving yourself permission to do so is where exceptional things happen.

You. Are. Exceptional.

It's time to live your exceptional life. No excuses.

I invite you to stand in your greatness and invoke the love, strength, passion and desire alive in you now, this very instant. Look, really look at your desires, your longings, the voice of joy and truly listen to what your body has to say. That deep quietness, waiting for permission to be heard. It's time to let the light in. Are you nauseous now? Keep going anyways.

Permission slips yield you power. They say "I can do as I please, I have the paper to prove it." You stand taller, braver and with more confidence. This is your YES.

Are you allowing yourself to live at the center of your own life? Whose permission are you waiting for? Instead of wiping the slate clean, recognize what's already there, hidden, waiting to be given its next breath. There will come a time when your inner goddess will demand more of your attention. Listen to her. Dare to consider her words as your desires. For many of us, the yearning to express our desires creates a fear of what might happen as a result. Judgment? Disconnection? Shame? So we stay quiet, small, and silent. And full of resentment. We feed the poison. And it becomes more potent. This is a journey about risk, about authenticity and courage. You can't own your truth, desires, and sensuality without the courage to tell the truth and set sail into the unknown.

Pulling up my anchor and setting sail is almost always a result of conversations and interactions with my husband, Kevin. My leaps and bounds in courage, bravery and vulnerability are direct results of the mirrors he holds up to reflect my truth.

For the past 20 years together, he has never told me what to do. He has never given unsolicited advice. Just exemplified truth and integrity and bravery and courage. Pain had long been my driver, my muse. It took me down some dark roads. But it was not long lived. Kevin's actions and silent mentoring paved the way for me to finally give myself permission to let my light shine. The rewards I received from being driven by pain were no longer cutting it. I stood in choice: let fear of what others thought about me, my story, my disclosure, my truth, paralyze me and lower my anchor or set sail.

Here's the truth about truth:

"I can let it confine me

Define me

Refine me

Outshine me

Or leave it behind me."

-Unknown, but Very Wise Author

And let us not forget another wise man, Albert Einstein's words:
"We cannot solve our problems with the same think-
ing we used when we created them."

How often have you heard something similar? And yet these true words are so often ignored. I was trapped in a cycle of banging my head over and over and expecting it not to hurt. There is pain and fear, and yet we often stay in this place. Why?

Your comfort zone keeps you trapped in your ordinary state of consciousness. If you could have solved your problem this way, you would have solved it long ago. But you're still here, banging your head and looking at the same answers. You come up against worry, fear, blame, guilt - everything, but the truth.

Jumping this major life hurdle can only be achieved by a major shift in consciousness. By becoming laser focused on the flawed foundation - the messages and beliefs that have kept you hostage in the now - you not only expand the depth of your self awareness, but give yourself permission to feel your authentic desires and express them because that anchor or uneven foundation will be healed and shifted into a launch pad for what you really want.

How do you mount the insurmountable summit, the absolute discomfort of your worst fears?

Faith.

Faith - in taking the first step towards intimacy and sensuality on your terms without seeing the next step.

Faith - that you are not only capable but deserving of feeling your truest desires.

Faith - that your choice is the right choice. No further explanation needed.

Faith - that "it feels right" *is* right.

What is it going to take for you to shift out of your comfort zone and expand into your greatness, into love, into intimate connection, into **you**? What does it look like to let yourself be seen?

When I existed from a place of shame, I did not honor my vulnerability or let myself be seen. My fear of disconnection held me hostage from my authentic self and creating fulfilling relationships with others.

I knew there was a way out when I honored my bravery and allowed myself to feel, unapologetically and uncensored.

I finally gave myself permission.

Permission for what?

- To be myself

- To put myself first

- To feel and honor my desires on a visceral level

- To not censor my wants

- To declare my intentions for myself and love

- To be a mother AND a woman with children

- To keep moving forward, even though the answer was not always clear

- To feel vulnerable and trust my intuition

- To not numb myself out to the good and bad emotions with food, drama and control

- To know I am worthy of love because I loved myself first

I gave myself permission to be me.

All of me, a mother and a women with children and a wife and a lover and a nurse and an entrepreneur and a loudmouth and a brave soul.

All I deemed good and all I deemed bad.

All of me.

I would never have been able to have this profound shift in conscious thought if I had not found support and reconnected to my body. My catalyst for change was to find the intersection of fear and vulnerability within myself, my oasis of courage. The insight you need to capture the desire, the courage and the essence of your truth is living just below the surface and waiting to emerge.

"Those who restrain desire do so because theirs is weak enough to be restrained."

William Blake

How would you like to be seen?

When I opened up my heart to support, the shrinking stopped and expansion happened. Expansion into love, abundance, acceptance, courage and vulnerability.

I wake up every morning knowing how I want my day to feel:

Clear.

Free.

Luminous.

Sensuous.

Ease.

This is my truth, the sound of my soul, the voice of my desire. It's liberating to own it.

Hella-scary the first time.

The second time? Absolutely.

The tenth? Familiar and warm.

Your voice and truth is real. It's time to honor it.

Permission is the gateway to possibility. I like to call on my future self when I am not shining as brightly as I could or need that extra dose of courage to move me through a difficult situation. I would like to introduce you to my future self, I like to call her Desiree. She is confident, owns her voice, shines brightly in the world and is overflowing with desire to connect, be nourished and be free in her body. I beckon her when I need my cup filled a little bit more, or need a polish to shine brighter. Desiree always shows up when I need her, because she is a reflection of all I hold beautiful and desire for myself, which is already inside me.

Naming your virtues and truths make them more accessible. They are yours for the taking. There is always a constriction in your body when fear lives there. Fear that you can't control what's happening, that it's never going to change. So name it as fear, and breathe into it. Visualize the fear leaving your body with every exhalation.

When you have a challenge, the first thing to do is to get fully present. Because when all of you is here, when you are fully alive, you can see the opportunities and take advantage of them. We usually do the opposite, going into defense mode and check out, waiting for the world to change around us and then we come out of hibernation. But it's never the right time.

Whatever is coming up for you - resistance, fear, digging in your heels, excuses, lists of why-nots - are signs you are coming up against something powerful and strong. Maybe an old message, a value, a belief that no longer works for you is hindering your progress by keeping you in your comfort zone.

After mapping out your fears and limiting beliefs, go back and look at the real you. Your truth, your desires, the way you want to be seen in the world, the way you want to feel. Recognize that all these anchors in your limiting belief systems are the very things blocking that divine feminine power, sensuality and raw expression. Just like I do with Desiree, tap into the future you who is fully expressed and liberated. What would her sexual permission slip look like? Write it out. Share it. Again and again.

Sharing your desires in the form of your sexual permission slip is a powerful choice. It can move you out of another common concern, overwhelm and into a life of pleasure, passion and joy you have never known. Without it, you will be stuck on the shore of your fears and insecurities, and that, my dear sister, is not where you belong.

CHAPTER 3
VULNERABILITY

I'll show you mine

I HAVE A secret to share. One that has been weighing me down and holding me back from entering into my greatness and excellence: I only recently emerged from my fear. This fear that had dictated my life and my relationships. This fear that was all mine. After 38 years of hiding behind it, my fear was finally given an eviction notice.

The shift happened as I sat with my husband late one Wednesday night.

I said, "I have a secret to tell you."

His eyes were welcoming and concerned, as always, giving me permission to keep going. "My secret is that I operate from a place of fear every day—fear of success, fear of failure, fear of judgement, fear of my truth and how powerful it is (so much so that I may not be able to stand it). It manifests as a force; an energy that visits me at night and churns up my doubts and insecurities for the day ahead." I said, "It's time to let it go because it's exhausting being me."

So he left me to my devices and I got out my sage to smudge

myself and the room of my fear—every dark corner, every hiding spot, every inch was cleansed. Every dark corner was exposed, the deep recesses of my memory, the tight spot in my abdomen that grows tighter as I get more scared. Everywhere.

After opening up my sliding door to the frigid air, I declared *"It is time for you to go now."*

I stood there for a good 10 minutes and knew the instant that it left.

The instant.

The fear, the weight, the sadness—all gone.

Scary? Yes.

Necessary? Yes.

Optional? No.

Giving away power of any kind is exhausting. Stop doing it.

I allowed my desire to spring forth. I owned it, and now it's mine; all the passion, expansiveness, worthiness, clarity and vibrancy. All mine. I sat there emotionally naked and vulnerable and it was shit scary, but necessary. It was different this time. The anticipation of future triumph and success prevented me from turning around to once again be guided by my past.

Just to cement the release, the expansion and emergence, I felt a calling to burn my old journals. Destruction is necessary to create space for the new, the brilliant, the truth to expand into. My sensual truth is not small. It requires space. It will no longer be contained. I had kept the journals to reference just how much progress I had made in my life. The last review revealed I had been essentially writing the same thing over and over for 20 years: I was desperate to be heard.

"Please listen," written over and over again; and my call, unheeded.

Ignored and deferred, looked over by the most important people in my life, my calls went unheard—so I grew louder, thinking I would be heard that way. No. I seethed and swallowed my rage, essentially ignoring its message and power. My growing anger, acting out, and rage always met with judgment, shame, dismissal as *just a phase, and silence.*

Silence. It was deafening. Did I matter?

In retrospect, I let not being heard define me and my actions. As I sat in my emotional nakedness, I was struck with expansion into what I could become; struck by communion, and clarity of who I truly am.

I was also exhausted by the releasing of the toxic emotional residue that was clogging my body with guilt and shame and fear about how success looked—and it certainly was not anything akin to anything I resembled. The fire burned hot as my hands glided over the soft leather of my journals for the last time, before they became ash. The emotionally charged writing of a dismissed child escaped from the pages.

Done.

Some burst into flames while others were a slow steady burn.

I reveled at the drama unfolding in my little wood stove. The result? The wisdom of my body (long ignored) kicked in with a kick-ass case of laryngitis; deeming me incapable of speaking.

Coincidence?

I think not.

Like purging the body of infection, I was letting go of all that no longer served me. This was my release and the evocation of my truth; the light, and the heat evoked my light and passion as I emerge from it exquisitely, beautiful, disarmed and of service as *me*. It was a process of purification and of celebration; to destroy old messages and reflections was to create space for me and my heart's musings—my truth; a space to lean into passion, and true intimate connection.

Today, my success and story are defined by my truth and my passion. Every choice I make is based on how it resonates in my body, my heart, intuitively. Sometimes my decisions have no reasoning or logic behind them, but I simply know. I reward myself for trusting my intuition, and in the first week of this practice of self trust, I had seen enormous prosperity and abundance in my life, my relationships, my children and my business. I needed to step into my greatness in order to see the rewards. In order to be heard, I needed to listen to myself, my intuition and my family by deconstructing messages and filtering them through love—pure and simple.

I was everything I admired and loathed and wanted. I reframed the perceived flaws into positives:

My "extra" 10 pounds? They made me an hourglass shape, which I think is damn sexy.

My nearsightedness? I am the proud owner of many pairs of fierce spectacles which I would not trade for any laser correction ever. My glasses are part of me, my brand.

My depression? I made it through two rounds of brutal postpartum depression and would not trade it for the world. This is where my journey to clarity began. I am grateful every morning to wake up and be authentically me.

Elise is a 35 year old mother of four who is rediscovering herself again after motherhood and trusting the voice in her heart instead of her fear.

I was at a meeting, and it was explained to me that the voice of fear and negativity is not me, and how to tell the difference between what is me and what is that fear. The voice that is not me is mean and shoots me down and tells me things like I can't and shouldn't, and that I am not good enough, I'll never figure it out, and why is this time any different?

When I hear that voice, instead of agreeing with it and believing it, I ask my heart if that's the truth and I'm surprised at how easy it's been to differentiate between the two, voices, even with just that little bit of clarity.

An example: I set a two week goal of losing 2 pounds. After two weeks, even with family issues and a cold, I stepped on the scale and actually exceeded my goal. I immediately was excited and celebrated and looked at myself in the mirror. Immediately, the voice came in and said, "stop celebrating about such a small thing, it's only 2 pounds. Maybe you didn't even lose it, maybe you just had a big poop since last time you weighed yourself. You may have lost it this week but you're just going to gain it back."

Then I realized that it wasn't me talking and I looked at myself in the mirror and smiled at myself for longer than 7 seconds and listened to my heart. I exceeded my goal and that's a good thing.

When I had that moment of realization, my body felt empowered, in control and kind of like butterflies in my tummy. Usually I describe butterflies in my tummy as anxiety, but this was different. It was a good feeling. Effervescent, like a 7-up soda. It was a happy bubbling. I got to control how that conversation went. Usually it was that negative inner voice that takes control, but I squashed it. The energy, enthusiasm and power came from deep inside of me, just deep. Beautiful. It has always been there, I just didn't know that I had the power to control those conversations. It might be deep but it's not far away or hard to get to. It's there whenever I need it, it just comes from a deep place. When I hear that negative voice, something goes click and I say I'm not going there, I go deep.

When I made the choice to listen to my real voice, my soft silent knowing chose awareness over the negativity I was hearing in my head. That voice doesn't come from a place of joy so that's how I know it's not real. Simple. It doesn't seem like it should be that simple, so that's why I've never done it.

I'm way more powerful than I thought I was. That voice has been talking to me for years and I did not know that I knew how to silence it until I was made aware that I get to choose. Now I'm in control of my thoughts and how I respond to things. I get to choose joy, I get to choose to listen to the language of my heart. That comes from deep within.

Without those negative thoughts, I am me. It also forced me to realize that I was living in a way that I wasn't meant to. I was covered in 40 pounds of not me. I was not me in that body. I was definitely not supposed to be numbing my life with alcohol as often as I did. I was not supposed to be feeling unhappy with my t family. With awareness, I realized that I didn't like living that way. I learned how to use my heart's voice to help me be me. I have big plans for the year ahead and I have taken steps to get me closer to my goals. My desire fuels me.

Let your desire fuel you, my love. But before you do, be vulnerable enough to shake off that negative inner voice as well as the fear and shame that try to dim the ferocity of your sensual soul and from there your beautiful desires can take root in fertile soil.

CHAPTER 4

TELLING YOUR STORY AND THE VALUE OF YOUR VOICE

"When we deny the story, it defines us.
"When we own the story we can write a brave new ending."

Berne Brown

BETWEEN GUILT, SHAME and fear, desire is a tough place to get to. It's not about which truths need to be given a voice, but rather which lies you are upholding as truths. It's time to find your desire, give it a voice and start living fully present. Naming your desires, your dharma, your purpose and path allow you to not only see the transition ahead, but also see the steps needed to move through it without sabotage.

Tending to your desire garden brings clarity and freedom to move through transitions. Fearlessly confront whatever stands in the way of your awakening. Watch the truth burst out. Trust your inner guidance and don't worry about getting it right. Writing your story allows you to own it. Connect to your own voice, your own passion and live that desire in your lifetime. Only you can write your story. Don't let someone else hold the pen.

Your sensual story has served you well. It serves many purposes in your life. Some of these purposes are beneficial, some are not. These stories are engrained in your values and beliefs and are often seeded in childhood experiences. Your story serves to keep you alert for future pleasures, to keep you safe, to honor and maintain your boundaries.

Everyone's story will be uniquely personal. I'll start with mine:

My story begins in elementary school.

I knew by the age of eight years old that I had been taught to be responsible for the happiness and the well-being of others. At this point, I did not realize the deficit that would occur in terms of fueling my own life, my own happiness and fulfillment. If there is a medal for busy-ness I would've won it. I carried on through my life being responsible for the happiness of my friends, my family, my coworkers. Every relationship that I had encountered always left me giving and giving and giving. I have done a tremendous amount of work to heal my past struggles and even though it was difficult, I am grateful for,the relationships I have with my family now.

I knew there was something off and I could not figure out what it was. I knew there was something missing. I also knew that this feeling of overwhelm, of fearfulness, of feeling stuck was not how I wanted to live my life. It wasn't until I met my husband, Kevin, that things started to fall into place. He was and still is a free spirit. He showed me what it was like to live truly and deeply in each moment. What I had not realized until this point was that I had been living a very superficial life. Within months of meeting him, I was living more impulsively and freely. I could taste a freedom I had never known. We would be on a plane to Mexico within 24 hours of deciding to actually leave. We were hedonistic and impulsive but underneath it all, it was pure fun. We were constantly seeking pleasure and new worlds started to open up for me.

It was an awakening. I was returning to Her, my true self. But there was one big obstacle on the horizon. We thought, "hey, if we have this much fun playing with each other, let's get married and build our family!" and so we did with the intention of expanding our potential for play and our potential for pleasure.

Our first baby came in 2005, a beautiful baby girl named Sophia. She was the light of our worlds and I took it fully upon myself to be her mom to do everything I could for her; to be responsible for her happiness, her health and well-being. What I did not realize was I had carried these false beliefs from childhood that I was completely responsible for her happiness, on top of everything else. It was to the detriment of my friendships, my relationships, my marriage and my own personal health.

I lost myself in motherhood. I forgot how to be a friend, wife and sister. Caring for Sophia was all I did. I defined myself solely as a mom. My return to Her had come to an abrupt halt. I had this false belief that I could not be a mother and be a sexual being. I could not be a mother and be open to pleasure because I dedicated every waking moment to my new baby.

Life had transitioned and I had not kept up with it. I was scared. I was fearful and hid inside my comfort zone. Inside, I was suffocating against the walls of my comfort zone. I needed to move, but again there was a feeling of overwhelm, fear and feeling stuck. I had lost the traction I had gained and couldn't even see where to take the first step. I didn't know what to do and that was the point where I completely bottomed out.

Within months of my daughter's birth, I was diagnosed with postpartum depression and treated with antidepressants as well as weekly counseling and group therapy with other women. It was at that point, I had my first glimpse into real vulnerability, the excruciating but necessary portal to expand my comfort zone. I surrounded myself with women in similar circumstances who grew tired of doing it all on their own and didn't have the language to ask for support. Women, with the pressures of the world on their shoulders, who were deeming themselves as failures against their unrealistic expectations as first-time moms, not knowing why or how or what to do. The only constant was that everything changed from minute to minute.

The consistent message that flowed from each one of my supporters and group members was this: *If I do not fill my own cup no one will fill it for me. I am responsible for my happiness, my well-being and my health.*

So I did it. I took my own advice and started filling my own cup. Over my 35 years, I had tapped out all the sources of perceived joy that I thought were there and then I was reminded by my gentle loving husband that I'd forgotten how to play. So I thought, "*why not, there's really nothing left...*" and when I dove back into play, what I discovered was that pleasure was fuel for me. I had just gotten out of practice and forgotten that along the way. I realized that this journey wasn't about becoming anything, it was about unbecoming everything that isn't me so that could be more of who I am and who I was meant to be in the first place. I am a pleasure seeker out redefining hedonism on my terms. I had allowed the role of mom to be bigger than me and as a result I let my sensuality die. Once I took time out of my to do list and started focusing on my *to be* list, my cup started filling up.

I got clear on what I wanted to be and it just kept filling itself up. I wanted to be free. I wanted clarity. I wanted to be luminous. Sensuous. Golden. Lit up. All of these feelings were on lockdown when I tried to fill the cups of others. I opened myself up to a sisterhood and they supported me as I allowed pleasure to fuel me through my erotic awakening. Little did I know how much I would need it with what was about to happen.

August 10th, 2004 started like any other day, but it was a special day. My birthday. I was freshly 34, excited to start my journey into motherhood for the second time. I was three months pregnant and had an ultrasound to date the baby's birth a few days earlier. I had made it through. Earlier in the year, I had been pregnant and went for my ultrasound, only to be met by the radiologist who said "there is no heartbeat. I'm sorry." Today was a new beginning, a new year, a new baby. It was fantastic. I was anxious heading into the ultrasound a few days earlier, as my previous experience was so painful. This time, the tech scanned my belly, and took the usual measurements and sent me on my way.

I spent the morning with my 4 year old daughter and we had a beautiful tea party, swung on swings, had a nap and spent the afternoon getting ready to go out for dinner with my husband once he got home from work. I remember the dress I was wearing: it was a new maternity dress that grew as I grew with small black and white flowers. I had a small belly by then, I had shown much earlier this time. I felt vital and whole and purposeful and feminine. Oh, so feminine. I was born to do this, to be a parent. My daughter was amazing and we had been studying all of the pregnancy books and measuring her soon to be born brother against walnuts, watermelons and peaches. We were all lit up. The pregnancy and subsequent parenting process of my daughter had been an intimate bonding experience between my husband and myself. We had a fantastic relationship and a baby added to our intimacy and brought us closer than ever before.

The phone call came at 4:30 pm. I was dressed up for my birthday dinner and sitting on the edge of my bed, lacing up my sandals in the warm heat. It was my midwife, Margaret. "Hi Lesley, I have your ultrasound results here in front of me." I immediately interjected, "Oohhh, let me guess, it's a girl, right? I can just feel it in my body. I just know it's a girl." Silence. "Margaret?" I repeated her name several times, "are you there?" A deep sigh on her end, my pulse sped up. My intuition screamed something was not right. Thoughts were spinning in my head and coming at me like a snowstorm, a whiteout. I couldn't think straight. "Margaret, what's happening?" I repeated.

"Lesley, there was no heartbeat. I'm sorry."

It hit me hard. I wanted to blame her. Why didn't the radiologist tell me, isn't that what they do? Why on my birthday? Why me? Margaret's voice interrupted my thoughts, "Lesley, I know you have been through this before, would you like to have another d&c? I can book that for you as soon as possible."

"Yes," I numbly mumbled.

"Okay," Margaret said, "What is your birth date?"

"Today, it's today. This is my gift today. This fucking sucks."

Silence again.

"I'm so sorry, Lesley, to have to share this news today, I'm so sorry."

We finished up the logistics and hung up, then I let the tears come. They were loud and guttural and primal and painful and they didn't stop. I slipped to the floor from the edge of the bed I had been perched on and cried my heart out. At this point, I felt the lightest touch on my head from my sweet Sophia, who kneeled down next to me and just held me. She didn't say anything, my 4 year old angel, just held me and patted my head. When I was finally able to compose myself enough to to speak, she spoke first, "Is my baby sister an angel baby, too, mommy? Like my other sister?"

I nodded my head yes. "Yes, she is, my lovely. I'm so sad right now, I'm not sure what to do." So we sat in silence until my husband came home a few minutes later.

He came in the house, loud and excited about our evening out, bounding up the stairs two at a time, "Where are my girls at?!" He appeared in the doorway, his face red from exertion, smiling ear to ear, arms outstretched with flowers, ready to deliver a love bomb to us. I'll never forget his face. He just knew. My daughter and I sat in a puddle of tears on the floor and he just knew. It was Sophia who spoke first, breaking the silence; "Mommy's baby died, Daddy. She's an angel baby now." He went limp, and the cuddle puddle grew bigger. This man, with such enormous love for his family, shattered. It was a moment, I'll never forget.

We did go out to celebrate. I remember being in the restaurant, but not in my body. Self deprecating thoughts ran through my mind: *I've failed myself, my body, my family, my husband. I can't get this right, how did this happen again? I don't ever want to get pregnant again. I'll just look into adoption.*

The pain of losing a child was too much to consider. I felt like a failure as a woman, as a person and couldn't see my way out of it. *How could this happen to me and my husband again? What's wrong with my body? Why can't I do this right? I was born to do this. Everyone else seems to do it, why not me? Will he still want to be with me, if I can't provide a child for him? He's done his part, it's time to do mine and I can't. I should know how to do this, I was born to do this. So why can't I get it right?*

The thoughts came fast and furious, like a snowstorm of shame and disappointment and fear. I was so scared. I never wanted to go through that pain again. Ever. It would take some big bravery on my part to even consider trying to get pregnant again. I felt like I wouldn't survive any more losses.

Sourcing out support and filling my own cup carried me through the next five years of tumultuous ups-and-downs including two back-to-back miscarriages and then after giving birth to my beautiful second child, I was slammed again with postpartum depression. But this time was different. I was in charge of my happiness and filling my own cup. I knew how to feel nourished, lit up and clear and free. The key was to tap into my pleasure as a fuel source. I shattered my false belief that I could not be a mother and be a sensual and sexual woman in the world simultaneously. I knew the familiar pull of the feminine from when I first met my husband. I knew the familiar sway and feeling that came with finding my feminine sensual flow and it was re-surging again. I could feel it and taste it. I intuitively knew I was returning to Her. Are you ashamed of your story? Your pitfalls? Your own squiggly lines? Is that the story you have attached yourself to? Instead of recognizing your falls as something of purpose, are you allowing shame to frame your story.

Berne Brown says, *"Shame is the unattainable and conflicting/ competing expectations about how we are supposed to be."*

Shame is all about disconnecting from our bodies, our true selves, ultimately ignoring our intuition which is attached to the bodies we are disconnected from. The solution? Get back into your body. Stop living in the expectations in your head. Begin to re-familiarize yourself with the sensations of fear, love, joy and shame when they arise in your body. Decide what stays and what needs to pass through and out the other side. Not allowing shame to pool and live in your body creates more space for love, pleasure and true intimacy to reside. Notice how different fear and love feel at a somatic level. It's up to you how much space you want to create for pleasure and joy to live within yourself.

"To realize one's destiny is a person's only obligation."
Paulo Coelho, The Alchemist

I invite you to explore your sensual story as a way to view how you see your sensual life, today. Your story creates a space for you to safely explore your attitudes, beliefs, experiences and values as they show up for you. Once you realize the lens in which you view your story, ask yourself, is this the lens I want to move forward with? Are my attitudes, beliefs, experiences and values serving me? Or keep-ing me stuck?

Journal on this:

Who do I think I should be?

Who have I been trying to be?

What false story have I been telling myself?

How has this story blocked my truth?

Write your sensual story. Recall your first memory of sensuality and pleasure. Just let go and free write, stream of consciousness style. See what arises. Sometimes it is painful, sometimes it is freeing.

Write about how you discovered yourself as a sensual person in the world.

Where did you learn about pleasure?

What was your first gut reaction to the word "sex"?

Writing your story is another important way to share yourself with the world. It is healing to be able to share your story and be witnessed. To be able to share your sensual story is about giving yourself permission to give it a voice.

Feel ready? Overwhelmed? Guess what? We all start before we are ready. We all feel not strong enough, ready enough or prepared enough to begin the journey - but we do. We take the big leap. No one starts the journey knowing all the answers.

Writing your Sensual Story:

Take an hour, create some space and write YOUR story. Not the fantasy you want it to be, but how it is now. This moment. Consider writing about your gender, growing up, your first and last sexual experiences. How you felt about them. What are your family beliefs around sex? Where did you learn about sex and sensuality? What you believe about your story. Your current relationship or past relationships. How did you show up sexually? What did you believe about how you showed up? Who were your sensual teachers? What is your experience around pleasure, power and orgasm? Write. I'll wait.

Now? Go do something really nice for yourself. What makes you feel great? Go do that. Refill your love tank. When you're ready, come back to your story and we'll keep going.

Telling your story is deep work. It is examining the roots of who you are as a sensual person.

A loud chatty voice that tells you your story is unimportant and even shameful is not your intuition. This is your head voice, your ego speaking out. The ego, this voice sounds and feels so much like you that you believe it is you. And it guides so many freaking decisions. You think you are telling yourself the truth. Stop believing this voice. Change happens through love, starting with you.

Your story is framed by your experiences and the value you place on those experiences. Imagine there are four pairs of glasses on the table in front of you. Each pair represents something different. The first pair is your attitude towards life. You view your life experiences through the lenses of your attitude towards it. Same goes for your beliefs, experiences and values. These form your unique point of view from which you view life and write your story.

Attitudes

If you are using your sensual story to build intimacy, you are on the right track. A friend may share that she was sexually assaulted in her lifetime. You may use this opportunity to share and disclose your experience with her, to build intimacy and connection. If you shroud your experiences in shame and secrets, this attitude will only serve to sever any intimacy.

Beliefs

This is a big one. All of our thoughts are neutral until we attach a belief to them. Byron Katie, the creator of The Work, defines beliefs this way: "A thought is harmless unless we believe it. It's not our thoughts, but our attachment to our thoughts, that causes suffering. Attaching to a thought means believing that it's true, without inquiring. A belief is a thought that we've been attaching to, often for years." I highly recommend doing exercises found in *The Work* to question your beliefs and the thoughts you have created out of them.

Experiences

Your life experiences shape how you view others. Each experience you have contributes to the lens in which you view the world. We bring our experiences to each interpersonal encounter. Sometimes this is helpful, sometimes it shows the seeds of assumptions.

For example, my first intimate experience with another human being was at 14 years old. It was not consensual and it was not violent. But it was still non-consensual. This could have set the stage for a lifetime of fear based intimacy and control issues around sensuality and sex.

Values

It is important to reflect on any concepts of morality and superiority you may be using in your story. Subliminal messaging and expectations of others may bring forth certain emotions when you hear them. Do your values reflect your story? Are they helping you move forward in your life and relationships? Or holding you back?

This is big work.

Congratulations, sister. You are being brave and diving in deeper. Big breath. Big love.

What themes emerged from your story?
Beliefs? Values?
Write them here.

Do they still serve you? Are they serving your highest good, your truth?

Yes? Fantastic. Frame them, keep them.

No? Time to ditch them and replace the beliefs. So we're going to jump back into *The Work* here.

The Work by Byron Katie is a series of questions about a specific belief that deconstructs the thoughts we have around beliefs. It is comprised of 4 questions:

1. Is it true?

2. Am I absolutely sure that it's true?

3. How do you react, what happens, when you believe that thought?

4. *Who would you be without the thought?*

When you feel fear, the challenge is to distinguish between a true threat and coming up against the edges of your comfort zone. So how do you distinguish between the two?

There are trolls, the voices in your head that don't belong there but occupy whole lot of space and airtime. Troll Taming expert Kimberly Linn Pollard has the answer:

"The easiest way to tell the difference between your intuition cautioning you and your trolls is to know your body. What does it feel like when your intuition is talking? My intuition feels centered around my torso, and I always feel sure and grounded when I listen to it. Even if the message I'm getting is a sense of foreboding, I still feel strong and connected. On the other hand, when the fear is coming from your trolls' attempts to hold you hostage, you'll feel very differently. My biggest clue is when I feel like my energy is buzzing frenetically around my head, I can't focus or be still. I feel panicky and out of control. Once you've determined the source of the fear, then it's just a matter of choosing what you're going to do about it. You can change your plan, put extra measures in place, seek out support, or ignore the fear altogether. Whatever you choose, remember that you are stronger than you think, and perfectly capable of handling whatever comes your way."

What are you chasing to fill the emptiness? Is it elusive? What makes you feel expansive? What do you need to say YES to? Who are you when you say YES to your intuition? The more you trust your intuition, the closer you get to the core of your desires. So rewrite your story, clean out what no longer serves you, lean into your divine knowing, and free fall into your desires.

CHAPTER 5
CREATING SPACE FOR DESIRE

*"There is no passion to be found in playing small - in settling
for a life that is less than what you are capable of living."*
Nelson Mandela

*"Waking up to who you are requires letting go of who you
imagine yourself to be."*
Alan Watts

YOUR DESIRES DESERVE space, my sister.
Every desire deserves to have life breath blown into it
and expand into its place in your life. Your true essence,
your life force is born out of the oxygen you nurture your desires
and longings with. What needs to be given less space, less breath,
less importance? Start there.

I'm betting you have heard this before: positive self-talk increases
your odds for happiness, joy and positive outcomes. It truly works
for me, along with gratitude and appreciation for what is right in

front of me. Ending the struggle to become something other than who you are is exhausting. There is another way.

Unpacking your sexual shame and embarrassment can be made easier with positive self talk. Then you get to the point where you cannot be objective about the next step; the scarcity of money, time and resources creeps in. This can make you feel disconnected from your body and your desire to exude sensuality from every pore and truly feel alive.

Are you feeling trapped by life? Deep down you know there is more crap that you don't know how to articulate and that keeps you stuck. As women, our cultural inheritance tells us to care for others and put them first, THEN take care of yourself with the remaining scraps of time and energy. Who is this woman? She is successful by most measures - children, job, home - but is often in fear of her body, numbed out to her true essence. Sound familiar? It's time to reverse your thinking on this skewed inheritance. When you choose to invest in yourself first emotionally, spiritually, financially from a place of abundance, everyone wins. When you make choices to support your health, you win, and by extension your relationship, your partner and your family flourish.

Amanda is a 30 year old life coach who went through a massive health scare that made her journey back to herself a priority.

Before my hysterectomy, I bled for so long, I hated my uterus. She made me feel mad. I told the surgeon, "I want to break up with my uterus." The anger came out as withdrawal, a kind of isolation. I felt really bad all the time. I fell into a depression. I did not offer all of myself to the world, and my family. Withdrawing affected me deeply. I knew I wasn't having the life I could have. I was mad at myself. The resentment stemmed from never getting relief from bleeding.

I felt empowered to have chosen to have the hysterectomy at such a young age. I felt empowered that I didn't choose to suffer. My life now is different because I feel freer. I can sleep naked. I feel freedom. I self pleasure every day of the week. Nothing stops me. I'm freed up to be myself and let go of the anger.

Who am I? I keep going back to a rebirth. I'm not 100% there, but I'm becoming that woman. I do have to renegotiate balance every day. I still have some grief over the babies I can no longer have. I am Amanda, a living breathing soul who sometimes feels that just breathing is enough. Just being me is enough. I don't have to be anything, just me. I've been in a space medically with blood clots where I can barely breathe, so being present and safe with my breath is enough for me.

My journey back to myself began when I realized there was more to sensuality and how I could access other women through the internet and see how different their lives were compared to mine, like how they were living and following their desires, having the sex that they wanted, having the sensuality they needed, and I was like, 'whoa, I'm not getting any of that. Where's mine?' So I went on the journey and I didn't even know I was on the journey, but I now know that what started it was when I expanded my world from just sitting here at home to having friends on the net and watching their lives blossoming. I wanted what they had.

Now, I get along with my spouse, I found the calmness and harmony.

I started reading erotica and it filled me up. I gave myself permission to sell pleasure and play around with textures like silk. I grew up being taught that masturbation was wrong. I left that story behind and I gave myself permission to tell my husband that I was getting a sex toy in the mail and that he could join me or not. At that moment I felt brave, so brave.

A woman truly in touch with her desires is a powerful force. I believe you can embrace this vital force and I am confident I can guide you to connect to your vital life force by honoring yourself, your decisions and your desires.

What is the first step to making room for pleasure? Tell your story. You did that in the last chapter. Release its hold on you. As Brene Brown so eloquently puts it, *"Shame cannot thrive without secrecy, silence and judgment."*

Create a STOP DOING list, as recommended by Danielle LaPorte, life strategist and author of *The Desire Map*. A stop doing list creates space for more of what you desire to emerge.

I have been honoring my Stop Doing List and creating space for my Lotus to come into full bloom. It was one of the scariest, yet necessary periods of personal growth I have ever experienced. My life is rolling out in the direction it needs to and I am loving the journey, even if I cannot visualize the destination from here. I am trusting life, trusting me.

May 23, 1995 was when I first started to clear the way and make space for my desire.

I was a young 20 year old, fresh out of my first serious long term relationship with a very religious high school sweetheart. I saw a glimpse beyond the confusing and contradictory web of religion, dogma, pleasure and my happiness. I saw an insight of another way to be in the world. I had an energy bubbling up inside of me that was effervescent, fun and getting louder by the day.

My sensuality. It was big and loud and felt good, but I surrounded myself with this energy that said "Be as you are. Don't let this out. Women don't act this way, women don't feel this way." So I sat on it. And still it got louder and louder and louder.

In retrospect, my transition was full of irony. I would attend bible study with fellow churchgoers and then jump into my car and head out with another group of girl friends and go dancing at the bars. More like on the bars, on tables, on chairs. My body, my soul wanted freedom and it wasn't being found in bible study. Moving my body, being with my friends, feeling uninhibited, felt like ease, felt free, felt like me. But I continued to suppress it. I felt like I was walking between two worlds—one I should be in and one I wanted to be in. Ignoring my intuition for the past 19 years had turned me into a people-pleaser. And finally my journey to honoring myself had begun. I knew there was more to this life than bible studies and early bedtimes.

It was at this point that I began to define spirituality on my own terms. I knew there was a force or an energy, something bigger than me out there that had a plan for me. I knew I believed in a God and also in the magnetic green earth energy. It was in the earth energy that I connected to my divine feminine power, my *shakti* and I knew I was on my way to finding inner peace through honoring my power. And I knew it involved sex somehow. Who knew it would be my career?

Freshly liberated from the church, I jumped head first into my sensual self. I had a taste of different relationships, some a matter of hours, some months long. Men, women; there was no differentiation. I honored my heart and where it wanted to go. Some relationships were intense, some boring. I longed for physical touch, not just sexual touch, but physical affection and true passion.

That is what had been missing. Passion. Intense passion. How did that look?

My limited insight told me this:

May 23, 1995
Dear Diary,

How love looks:
(None of them are deal breakers but all of them would be excellent)

1. Very outgoing.

2. Encouraging.

3. Adventurous. *(pretty insightful so far)*

4. Has to drive a Jeep

5. Will dance in the headlights of said Jeep with me.

6. Affectionate, to give me all the touch I need all the time.

7. Have goals.

That was it. Nothing too lofty.

Fast forward to 2016, and I am a sensuality coach with a thriving practice, registered nurse, sexual health educator, have been passionately married 13 years and have two young kids whom I adore.

I was cleaning up my daughter's room when I found my old diary in the back of her toy chest. My heart fluttered as I opened it. It was a paradox in cursive. The first few pages were biblical scriptures from bible studies and the last few pages are a detailed description of how I fell in love with my husband.

I thought: Should I share this with him? What would he think?
My body said YES, so I did.

My husband was quietly reading in the early evening and I perched next to him, as I always do, head on his shoulder and snuggled into his broad ribs and said "Look what I found, my old diary from 20 years ago." And I started to read.

I read slowly. Scripture at first, the sadness of a death of a high school friend lost too soon, the slow death of a relationship choked and suffocated by religious dogma and expectation, the excruciating pain of a breakup and being replaced.

Then I came across my list with my appraisal of how my husband-then-boyfriend fared...

I read on.

May 23, 1995. How love looks:

> *I got flutters in my stomach as he leaned in. There was that look again. That-I-can't-take-my-eyes-off-you-look.*

It was like he was looking into my soul.

1. Very outgoing? Yes, social and private in beautiful balance.

2. Encouraging? Endless encouragement.

   So far, so good

3. Adventurous? Yes, he has joined me on spur of the moment trips to Mexico and Oregon with less than 24 hours' notice. "Hmm, it's Tuesday. How do you fancy Puerto Vallarta this Thursday, my lovely?" I'd say. "Perfect,"he'd respond.

4. Has to drive a Jeep? Volvo station wagons are sexy right? Motorcycles built for 2, also a big thumbs up.

5. Will dance in the headlights of said Jeep with me? Yes, on one of our crazy roundtrips.

   OMG, I was getting goosebumps as I read it all aloud, my husband's eyes intent on my moving lips.

6. Affectionate, to give me all the touch I need all the time? My big learning with this came with learning each other's "love language", a program designed by Dr. Gary Chapman. Mine is, you guessed it, Touch.

7. Have goals? He is the only man I know who gained clarity on his career goal and achieved them in less than eight

months. He is currently on a journey of spiritual awakening and the vulnerability he exudes is so incredibly sexy.

(That will be the next book I'm thinking!)

A+.

Since writing my list 18 years ago, I have grown immensely as a woman and now define happiness and get to choose it every day by waking up in the morning and choosing to feel the way I want to feel, by engaging in activities that make me feel the way I want to feel. I am always at choice, every minute. I get to choose pleasure.

My subconscious chose that very moment, both of us leaning in, to reveal that it was not about what was on the list, it was the behaviors, actions and requirements that made me feel the way I wanted to feel—to find a partner that makes me feel adored, abundant, aroused, passionate, worthy and fully alive every day.

Jeep optional.

"Go inside and listen to your body, because your body will never lie to you. Your mind will play tricks, but the way you feel in your heart, in your guts, is the truth."
      — Don Miguel Ruiz, The Four Agreements

I often see women living by default with the repeated refrain of "I don't know what I really want, I'll just take what is left." Your desire is a powerful thing, one that has a capacity to allow you to live a life better than you ever dreamed. Tune into it, listen. Follow it. Pleasure heals. The state of arousal is the seat to every woman's power. Embrace your sensual flow, deeply integrating pleasure, play, and relaxation into every moment. Pleasure is the goal. Allow pleasure to re-inhabit your body.

Getting your sexual desire back doesn't have to be difficult or time consuming. It does, however, mean you sit down and take an honest assessment of why you don't desire sex. Once you figure it out, moving into a sex life that you look forward to is quite easy. Create space by giving up habits that no longer support you and make room for new growth.

I got in touch with my energy, my Shakti, and let the wisdom of my elders and inherent feminine voice guide my path. It's time to shed the shoulds and wake up to life as it was meant to be lived. Full out. Alive and awakened. Defined by you. It's time to say yes to personal truth and authenticity and reclaim your passion for life and your innate embodied power. It's time for an inner revolution.

What is the biggest risk you have ever taken? You know the shifts I mean; the moves and shifts that make you nauseated just thinking about them. They make you break out in a sweat and make you want to immediately distract yourself by checking your email again instead of keeping yourself focused on your inner workings and nudges. Do you allow your struggles to define you and your interactions in the world? Do they keep you in your comfort zone, just safe enough to keep moving forward? They raise their noisy heads at times when you least want them to but you have worked out a strategy to keep them quiet and hidden out of sight. It's almost easier to live that way; small, quiet and safe. Those are the results you will reap; small quiet and safe. Want something bigger? Can you handle your true desires?

For so long, our desires have been couped up; we have been conditioned and fed to believe what the greater good desires for us is more important that those desires bubbling up within us. That this - the shoulds, the box, the safe, the quiet - is what you want so you don't kick up a fuss to avoid unwanted attention and fuel the cycle of feeling unattractive and numb. Just conform and shut up? You don't want that.

What needs to be shrunk, destroyed, buried or removed altogether from your life and time to make space for your desires to emerge? Is it emotional care taking of others? Is it putting yourself last on your to do list? Is it making the kids lunches and not yours and living off caffeine until your 2pm self implodes with starvation? Making sure he has an orgasm first? Whatever it is, start there. Every day, do a little less of what you don't want to do and a little more of you do.

Surrender is the essence of the feminine. Because you can only feel love. Challenge your lifelong programming and fearlessly confront whatever stands in the way of your awakening. Loving yourself is important but accessing it through your heart, rather than your brain, is a different story. Does contentment make you nervous? Do you feel the need to uplevel once you have achieved 'this'? How do you celebrate your successes? Do you savour them or move on to the next item on your list? Savour the moment, relish yourself.

When I listened to my heart's voice, I reawakened myself to my truth. I gave myself permission to express the most sensual parts of me and learned to believe that there is nothing more beautiful than my truth. I was unbecoming my social programming, my lies, my fears and becoming more of who I was all along. Reclaim the nagging persistent feeling wanting to break through, trapped under generations of cultural inheritance and shaming.

The yearning, the longing for surface, for that first breath of air that says you have arrived, has been waiting for you. We've made space for you. We have destroyed that which no longer served us for your arrival. You have so much to teach us, and the learning has already begun.

Your wisdom, your longing, did not go unnoticed. It started as a whim, a nudge from the divine that "perhaps we should feel a bit more into this one" and you did. The journey to the surface is part of the magic. Now that you have tasted this air, sweet with anticipation, with readiness, with compassionate acceptance, you can no longer sink below the surface again. This is where you live now; alive, ignited, luminous and ready to break your personal freedom barriers.

You are returning to her. We are Wild Women. Find your true power in being you.

Truth: you in no way need to prove yourself to receive love, joy or connection. Being yourself is the ultimate treasure in life. It is also the scariest, most rewarding journey you will ever take. Your perceived cracks and flaws are not imperfections, rather glimpses of your radiance waiting for permission and pleasure to emerge.

Why do you deny those things that you know will enhance your life? Why do you deny your senses, intimacy, connection and pleasure? Ask yourself: what are you deserving of? What do you choose to let in? There is infinite room for love connection and joy, yet we limit how much we need. We need more. Scrubbing out the dark spaces and corners make room for more. Make the room for it to enter and reside. Give yourself permission for your pleasure to take up space.

Say yes to one of these things for it will surely seep into all the other areas. Let's say pleasure. What if you said yes to every single experience of pleasure that came by in the next week?

Yes to trying on cashmere, without getting into the story of why you can't afford it.

Yes to taking a second inhale of the heady spring bulbs emerging from the earth, yes you have time for that.

Yes to intimate connection and intimacy with another human. This may mean the most erotic eye gaze you've ever had or perhaps writing how your partner makes you feel in your skin and reading it aloud to them.

Try it. 24 hours. I dare you to stop.

Pleasure is all around you now. It's about slowing down and using your erotic energy as a portal to your personal power. How willing are you to take emotional risks? What is your default behavior when you are emotionally exposed? Do you bite back, lash out, or melt further into vulnerability to see the claws, the messages and the fears truly keeping you at a standstill?

Your internal space has to be given the same level of respect and diligence as our external space. This means constant ongoing, sorting, de-cluttering, space-scrubbing, sorting through the dark corners of the mind and mining out the cobwebs and residue of shame, guilt - the feelings that represent choosing fear over love.

You have everything you need to experience the most sensual version of yourself today, right now. It's all in you - the confidence, the language, the self-assuredness, the voice of your desires. Your pleasure is alive and well, however you may be out of practice expressing it. Your desires may be hidden and obscured behind old messages, emotional clutter and outdated expressions of fear. Your desires deserve space. You have a choice to remove the clutter and shine light into the dark corners and experience just how much pleasure your life can embody.

What's holding you back from the most sensual version of yourself? What's holding you back from fully owning and being in alignment with your desires? You. Your thoughts and values. Your inhibitions are very much tied into your sensual story that you wrote in Chapter 4.

What are the themes that you extracted from your story? What are the messages? Rewrite them here.

This is where the excavation begins. What do you want to create room for? What needs to fall off the end? What is taking up space that could be occupied by more sensual moments? Only you know.

Ask yourself:

Do you need to...
say No more often?
say Yes more often?
Re-examine your boundaries around emotional care taking?
To establish time in your calendar just for you?

What do you...
Need and want to learn more about, purely for interest and intrigue?
Need to get clear on to bring you more joy?
Give yourself permission to say "I'll think about it and get back to you."

Your desires are your compass. They direct you towards more pleasure and joy and love. Do you want more pleasure, joy and love? Yes? Fantastic. Keep going.

What do you want more of in your life? Truly? This is your desire speaking. Declare your desires. Let the universal energy know what you are seeking. Be clear. Be specific. Let us know. Tell a girlfriend. Be witnessed in your desire seeking. You may find a fellow desire seeker on the same path. You're never alone in this journey. Your beliefs define who you are and how you choose to show up in the world. When you get really clear on what it is you believe and create safe spaces for freedom in full expression, your bliss and pleasure get activated

Chapter 6
Femininity

"The feminine fire is a primordial elemental force that is powerful beyond our wildest imaginings.
It is, in fact, power itself."

Teri Degler

YOUR FEMININE NATURE is always in flow. Often we encounter blocks and jams in the flow and become accustomed to this new reality. All the while, our powerful feminine essence, our life force, keeps building behind the blocks and awaits the destruction of obstacles to move through again.

The dance of the masculine and feminine are always in flow, dancing and interconnected with each other. The feminine is what really allows us to get in tune with what we really want and then start attracting and manifesting what we need to make it a reality. It is in constant flow with our masculine which can help us take that focused action in alignment with what we truly desire When we respect and understand both energies, we save a lot of energy and move closer to the results we are looking for.

Step out your sensual shame and into your erotic feminine power. Your feminine energy is your limitless source of inspiration, of vitality and of creativity. Your personal feminine power is tied up within you.

XTine Fine is the stage name of a 56 year old burlesque dancer who gave herself permission to express her sensuality when she was in character. And it didn't stop there - it extended to every other area of her life.

I am a woman that is bisexual and I hid it for many, many years. I went into my marriage as a straight person. In the past 10 years, I have had several sexual relationships with women. What brought it about was the death of my mother 10 years ago. She was killed in a car accident. It was so shocking to me that everything I knew before seemed different. I knew that I was married, but I did not consider it it cheating, more of a journey or an exploration, because I'd always felt shame regarding it and I knew it was something that I had to overcome. And when I came to terms with the fact that I was a bisexual and I love woman, I became a more empowered and sexy woman.

Seven years ago, I became a burlesque dancer. I did it as a challenge to my husband because I knew he wouldn't approve but I ended up loving all of it, the show, the creativity, the costumes. Our town had a yearly show and I developed a character in which I could express myself through and give myself permission to be over the top sexual and creative. My mom taught me how to sew so I make all my costumes, and choreography, with a live band I choose my own singer. It's my show. It's my imagination.

When doing burlesque, I'm at home in my body and empowered. It's kind of like when some people say they have negative self talk and talk themselves out of something, saying, "do I want to do this at my age?" When I hear that, I know that's my shame speaking. When I am going through the process of transformation into my character, whether it is practice, a photo shoot, rehearsals, making costumes, it keeps me in my body. I do something to invest in myself, like a show or boudoir photos every three months to keep my confidence up. I've given myself permission to be sexy and to carry myself with complete self-confidence. Whenever I do my pin up photos, there is always something in each photo that is significant, like including a red rose that is a symbol of my mom. They were my favourites.

Burlesque is my portal to accessing my sensual self. I love the art of tease, of reveal.

I desired freedom and I found it.

Feminine embodiment is about being in your body and getting out of your head. It's about being fully present and trusting your intuition and sensations in your body, without judgement. Just feeling them as they happen.

Stop the distractions and start being present. For some of us this is a real struggle, as it feels unsafe to us, to be alone with ourselves. Your body has so much wisdom. Once you feel safe and trust the inherent wisdom in your body, being fully present, amazing things happen. It's time to break up with external validation and approval. It's time to dump others' definition of your success. Time to take imperfect action.

There is no better time than now to invest in yourself. Now. Today. You will never be more ready than this instant. Making time for yourself is a beautiful way of nurturing your feminine. Too much yang energy, like working nonstop will leave you feeling depleted. Linear and in the box thinking leads to being stuck in the masculine. Modern living has dictated this linear thinking and separates you from your feminine glow. There are no coincidences or whims. Life shows us clues which are, in fact, gifts, but we miss them living in our head and not trusting our bodies. Asking yourself truthfully what do I want and what do I desire and having the patience to wait for the answers allows you to settle into your femininity.

It's time to cultivate curiosity, to break the mold. So much energy in Western culture is based on acquisition, the latest gadget, the newer, bigger, better. They are all diversions and distractions. This is not sustainable. Instead of looking externally, create your own success internally. Get out of your head and intuitively trust your body. Cultivate curiosity. Make pleasure a practice. It's about the reintegration of desire back into the core of who you are.

How do you nurture your feminine? It's slowing down, peering inwards, introspective honoring time. Come to know your feminine superpowers - intuition, sensuality and desire - as a powerful triumvirate of feminine energy. Feminine energy is about *being* instead of *doing*. It is rooted in self love and supported by intuitive action. It allows you to gently blow on the embers of your feminine energy. When the door swings open, pay attention to what you receive, hear and see.

Feminine energy is rooted in yin - receptive, fluid, intuitive. Yang is the active, focused, manifesting, and intellectual. When a woman learns to heal, transform and utilize her sensuality - her vital life force - she becomes a magnetic force. When a woman learns to source from yin energy, things shift to more pleasure and balance. Yang brings depletion, stress and exhaustion. It is a common and untrue belief that yang is the way to get things done. Shiva without Shakti is stagnant. Shakti without Shiva is chaos. It's a dance.

Shakti in its purest essence is divine feminine energy. Energy. It is what fuels us. Feminine energy is centripetal energy which spirals up from earth. It draws people in. It is irresistible energy. It's energy coming up from earth and spiraling through our uterus, breasts and tonsils and attracting those around us.

Shakti is divine feminine energy and is alive and well within you. It is in a constant interplay, a dance with the masculine, also known as Shiva. Both energies serve to balance each other, the masculine bringing consciousness and the feminine Shakti being creation.

We need a balance between the two to get in touch with our desires and fully live. When your Shakti energy is awakened and nourished, you shine. People notice. You are in alignment. You've got that je ne sai quois (RIGHT SPELLING?). You have this energy within you, you always have, since you were a child. Shame, fear, obligation and guilt are common ways this powerful energy can become squashed and lose its reverence.

Returning to Her literally means reclaiming your Shakti energy and living a fully awakened life. Shakti means to come home to yourself. As you are.

Drop into Shakti, connect and open up to it. It wants to flow freely. What does that mean for you recognizing your powerful feminine energy and how can you cultivate it? It expands awareness, opens into divine states of consciousness, opens your heart space. It may be instinctive, but if we don't nurture it or give it any value, it goes back into hiding, just like your creativity.

Creativity is inextricably linked to your sensual feminine power. It ebbs and flows, with cycles, with the tides and with life stressors. Tune in to the context of what is happening for you when your creativity emerges. What time of day is it? Where are you on your cycle, if you are premenopausal? What are your surroundings? What events have just happened? How have you nourished yourself?

As women, we tend to avoid creative shifts as they appear for three main thoughts:

1. everything is going so well, why shift?

2. what if it doesn't work out?

3. I'm scared about the unknown, the future.

When creativity wanes, it is usually a sign of lack of inspiration or a massive life transition that requires an upleveling. When mastery becomes tedious, and boring, it's another sign to uplevel. This is your opportunity to uplevel to another creative incarnation. Fear will crop up for sure, although it has no perspective. Its very job is to keep you safe and if its only option is to make up stories about how crazy your new perspective is, then fear will do just that. Easing up on your expectations will help you reach your creative goals. Taking it easy on yourself and being an observer of thoughts and ideas, instead of owning them, will keep you as objective as possible.

"I want to feel nourished, abundant, clarity, freedom, expansive. Can you do that?" These were my first words to my photographer friend, April, who was going to take some business shots for me. And some *other* photographs, too. The kind that made me nauseated just thinking about them. Those ones. The ones ladies my size didn't do. Or so I thought.

My hangup about visibility came up for me before I was even having the photographs taken. What did it mean to be seen? You're talking to a woman who didn't even get University graduation photos taken. I have lots of energy circulating around being seen, success and recognition. My shit, my gremlins asking me, "Who do you think you are?" More thoughts came up to the surface: *nobody wants to see this body, you're not a model, you want to that these photos to show whom?* The floodgates of shame and worthlessness opened wide and the deluge was messy. It was my mess, contained behind years of codependency, emotional abuse, emotional eating, low self-worth and wanting to be accomplished yet simultaneously invisible. My thermometer for success was set on low. And every time I wanted to raise it, I felt massive resistance. So I backed off.

All this surfaced before the lens cap came off. I had crafted an entire story about how bad the experience would be before we even began, about how I was a huge inconvenience to the photographer by being a burden on her time, resources, insulting her craft with my enormous thighs and belly folds. Boy, was I wrong. My lovely, feminine, Goddess photographer April arrived at my doorstep and I started sweating from nerves. We exchanged pleasantries about the nice dresses I had picked out, knowing quite well they would not be used for the entire shoot.

"What do you want to come out in the photos?" she asked. "What do you want to convey?"

"I want to feel nourished, abundant, clarity, freedom, expansive. Can you do that?"

"Yes. It's in you. I can help you capture it." At that moment, I mentally created a box to put my fears, insecurities and unworthiness into and gave myself three hours to ignore it. Just three hours. I told myself: *I can do this. I've got this. She's here for me.* I wanted to throw up at that very moment. But didn't. This is what expansion felt like and I wanted expansion.

We picked a sunny secluded location with a great mixture of light and shade, trees and grass. Being outdoors felt very freeing, nourishing and expansive, everything I wanted. *Keep going,* I thought, *you've got this. This is what you say you want.*

She took some stock business photos for me to use as a warm up, and then the time came. The time to take off my clothes. And be naked, like really naked. Nude naked. All the way. It was time for those photos. By this time, I felt like dry heaving and wanted to go reclaim my fears and unworthiness from the box — but I didn't.

Instead I dug deep, found my courage and stared down the lens of her camera with my soul, my bare breasts and my stretch marks exposed. I kept breathing and with each breath, drew in more of what I wanted to feel: clarity and abundance, expansiveness and freedom.

This was freedom. I had finally tasted it. April snapped away and with every click, I opened up further. Each breath, I released my fears and trusted her presence, her steadiness, her love. She lowered her lens and said "Are we done or are there any other photos you'd like to take?"

I swallowed, hard. I could feel that lump, that imaginary one that comes up when you don't want to say something, but know it needs to be said. The whole reason we were here. "Yes," I said, I want you to take photos of my vulva." There I said it! I waited for the "no" from April, but it never came. "Of course, I'd love to." She instructed me to sit, lay and crouch in certain ways in order to capture the uniqueness of my feminine flower. The best shot of the day looked like this: as I squatted in the grass, the sun came up over the horizon and it appeared as though the sun was shining from my feminine source, my yoni. It was an incredibly powerful photo and my favorite of the entire day. It glowed burnt orange and yellow and illuminated everything around it. On that day, in the grass, I finally returned to Her, to my source, my vitality, my sensuality.

I got back into my body. I trusted my body. Like a baby learning to walk, my body knew what it had to do. When I outsourced my expectations to others, I was living in my head. I was only living above my neck. I did not trust my body, this body that had carried me, that had kept me safe, that had birthed two babies, completed university, created thousands of beautiful orgasms, created these words for you, this same body. Since when did the package define the contents? I stopped living in my head and began to re-familiarize myself with the sensations of fear, love, joy and shame when they arose. I needed to firmly decide what stayed and what needed to pass through and out the other side.

As your courage grows, so does your momentum into fully embracing your truth on a soul level. What can you do to connect to your body today? One of my favorite ways is dancing, awakening my Shakti energy, the divine feminine goddess alive in all of us.

Dancing also activates your creative center, your harnessed sexual energy in your sacral chakra.

It's time to wake it up. I dare you to wake up your pleasure through dance, through movement.

Now.

I'll wait, take as long as you need.

How did it feel? Did you feel the sexual energy start to circulate and rise up in your body? It may feel foreign, but get to know it will be of great service to you if you let it.

Femininity is a great intimacy igniter in relationships. It is the fuel that fires the intimate connection in my 20 year relationship with my husband, Kevin. We are both in touch with our Shakti and Shiva energies and have created a safe space to explore them with each other:

He leaned in, my sweet Kevin.

"How are you feeling?" he said, earnestly.

I pondered, "Hmmmm, I've got some recognition, some vibrancy, some worthiness, and lots of passion going on. Feeling pretty switched on, I'd say."

"Whatever has shifted for you, keep going. It's very attractive. I like it." He smiled coyly and reached out to tuck a rogue curl behind my ear.

Ever since letting go of fear, the erotic energy and positive vibrations are flowing in my relationship like crazy. Like oozing from our pores. The air is heavy with acceptance and connection and love and passion.

Switched on.

Loving me.

Loving him.

Loving us.

The intimate connection is crazy hot.

So what happened?

We have always been very connected and it is amazing to think that we could take this intimacy, this connection, to another level.

The crazy-I-know-what-you're-thinking-right-now-crazy-and-you-didn't-even-open-your-mouth feeling.

The palpable connection.

The energy.

Presence.

The YES.

Your inner self is dying to emerge and fight against any more darkness or numb greyness. Every attempt to dampen Her spark, Her embers, is met with silent, but present opposition and She lets you know. Her voice is growing louder and louder and you can't ignore it anymore. It's time to send out the invitation. You know to whom, She's out there, waiting to receive it. Patiently. She has been waiting a long time for you.

Return to Her.

CHAPTER 7
SENSUAL SURRENDER

RECLAIM YOUR CAPACITY to be sensual for yourself and own it completely as the divine illuminated whole erotic sensual woman you are. Get deep down into the core of your sexuality in order to coax it out. Give yourself permission to delve into the fullness of who you are, to come into alignment with the frequency the vibrancy of who you are and boldly take up space.

I am a practicing sensualist, a person devoted to the physical, especially sexual pleasure. My own sensual awakening came in the summer of 1986.

The summer of 1986 was warm and bright and hot. The grass was dead and scorched in the summer sun. Newly christened into tweendom as an 11 year old, my birthday had just passed and I was doing what other 11 year olds do: spending everyday with my BFF. We had days-long sleepovers, shopping excursions with our $2 allowances and spent most days in her swimming pool. My hormones were raging and I remember the highlight of being at her house was getting to see her 15 year old brother every day. I dreamed about passing him in the hallway at night on the way to the bathroom, and watched him eat breakfast every morning while I pretended to eat. It was pure heaven. His name was Tony and I was in puppy love. He didn't particularly say much to me, or anyone else for that matter, but I could feel my cheeks flush every time I saw him. Sometimes he would join us in the pool with his friends which made for a fab day.

Early one August morning, my friend and I created our nest by the pool: books, pillows, towels, water, candy, and some shade. I dove in repeatedly and pulled my body out of the pool easily, onto the edge and crawled out. I did this over and over and over. Until I discovered the jets.

Oh, the jets. After a dive, I surfaced and made my way to the side of the pool. I put my hands on the cool tiles to pull myself up. It was then that I felt the pressure. The jet on the side of the pool had come into perfect alignment with my clitoris. Wow. The pressure was intense and I pulled away. And then returned to it.

"I'm tired, so I'll just hang out here for a minute, K?" My friend nodded in agreement. The pressure was causing my heart to beat faster, I could feel my pulse in my ears. There was a heightened sense of alertness in my body, like it was anticipating something, but I couldn't quite figure it out what yet. The intensity of the pressure and alertness grew and my head started to feel congested. I felt like I had to sneeze but couldn't quite make it happen, it was like being on the edge of a sensation, without fully experiencing it.

Then it happened. The sneeze-like feeling rolled over into a wave of what I now know to be an orgasm. My pupils dilated, my head turned into a complete fog. My escalated breaths stopped. My body rocked with pleasure and my fingers and toes curled. Instinctively overcome by pleasure, I let go of the side and slid under the water. It was otherworldly.

Disoriented, I took a deep inhale and swallowed a huge mouthful of water. I surfaced, sputtering and coughing, being pulled out of the pool by none other than the exquisite 15 year old Tony himself. "Holy crap! You almost drowned! Did you fall asleep? You were on the edge there for a long time!"

"Um , yeah," I murmured. My insides hungered for more. And

I dove back in, careful not to let go this time. I lived in that pool for the rest of the summer.

There comes a time in your spiritual journey when you have to let go of who you think you are, what you think you're good at and what you know about yourself. It is when we truly surrender and give over control to the divine that we truly find ourselves.

Sensual energy is the highest transmitter of creative energy. Sensual stimulation literally wakes us up. Pleasure is a powerful source of joy, vitality, self-expression and healing. Yet it is so stigmatized and shamed in our culture. Sensuality is the connective tissue of life. Art is creation materialized. Creative energy is a vital force in every person. It is the force that shifts the currents, the sails towards the ultimate destination. It is a potent energy. Women's sensual energy is the fuel that lights up a woman from within. Learning to access and utilize arousal is the beginning of wholeness. Arousal is the ignition switch to the female erotic engine.

Just ask Christina.

Christina is a 40 year old business woman who loves music. She has come to the point of surrender in her relationship to her sensuality:

> *I've come to understand that there are so many different things that sex is, and the primary one is a reflection of my relationship with myself. Another one is a reflection of my level of connection with my acceptance of my body. One of them is a connection with where I'm at in my life in terms of almost like a spiritual balance. Am I at a place where I am present and available in my relationship I that way?*

> *It's a reflection of emotional connection and intimacy, it's a reflection of evolving in my relationship in a way that is about this kind of mutual connection.*

When I think back to this time that it was this big scary act, and what it comes down to is the act of sex itself is such a beautiful sharing experience, but the things that makes it that and the things that get in the way of making it that are entirely different. It's not really about us at all, it's about me and where I'm at with it.

These beliefs about my lack of confidence physically or expectations of what I should be at physically in order to be desirable. Desirable isn't even the right term, I thinks it's that unconscious. I think it's like when I'm feeling in a good place with who I am, it's a natural outflow. Some of it, I think is honestly habitual. It's about just deciding to truly make a conscious decision that this is an important part of my relationship and I know once I say yes, I'm always in. I can honestly count on one hand how many times I've said yes and not been glad that I did. In these cases, I did not ask for what I wanted and in turn, I didn't get it. Sometimes the things that get in my way, it's almost like laziness, or the newest Netflix series, apathetic, I'd rather just tune out. It's a powerful experience to connect with someone on that level and honestly, sometimes there are things that feel easier than having that experience. Sometimes it's easier to opt out and then opting out becomes a habit, then your new normal.

When I want to get in touch with my sensuality, I use one of the tools Lesley gave me. Self pleasuring. Sometimes I connect with my own pleasure first and see where it takes me. That's really helped me to connect with my husband. Sometimes when I'm struggling with coming into alignment with my sensuality, I'll say it out loud. I'll say, 'I'm struggling with this right now' and the honesty builds intimacy between us, and allows him to support me and allows me to be honest and accountable. Yes, I do want this and I get to have a conversation with him about the impact of this power in our relationship. I am grateful for the conversations Lesley and I have had and how it's given me the freedom to understand how I operate as a sexual woman. I don't think our society really honours a personally pleasurable relationship with oneself. It is an incredible gift to give to yourself and your partner. I think it's actually communicated in the opposite way, like why would you do that if you have a husband, what does that say to your partner? It says I love my partner and it's important that we have this part of our relationship as a priority. It says I love myself enough to bring this most intimate part of me to my relationship.

Christine wiped the sleep away from her eyes and got a clear vision on how owning her sensuality would benefit her relationship with her partner. Ready to wipe the sleep away from your eyes and wake up? Settle in, be still and let her know you are here. Tell her, "I am here. I am here." Feel her essence arise within you. It is been sometime since you last connected, give her time to wake up and emerge.

"A personal legend is the reason you are here, it's a simple as that. You can fill your hours and days with things that are meaningless. But you know you have a reason to be here. It's the only thing that gives you enthusiasm."

Paulo Coelho

Why should you allow Her to emerge? Life demands to be felt, to be tasted in full. Yet we often don't have the skills to navigate being full in, so we opt out. Way out. And never grow. Imagine if you had the skills to play fully engaged, with all your senses, with your whole self, uncorked, uncensored, uninhibited. This is how life is meant to be lived. Where are you living?

It's time to come clean.

To tell the truth.

To feel the unfolding, to take ownership of the energy surfacing as your light shines brighter.

To come clean and face your desires, and to let yourself be truly seen. The chaos of our outer world is in direct proportion to how much you choose to ignore the shifts happening in our inner world. Perhaps your outer world has not caught up with the amazing shifts we are making towards greatness.

What are the most effective tools you can use to make your inner and outer worlds more congruent?

Acceptance

Know that others in our environment are a mirror for our personal growth. It's about acknowledging your own piece in the chronic, inflamed friction with a lover, a child, a co-worker. What can you do with this awareness and acceptance?

Forgiveness

Yourself first and foremost. Showing yourself empathy and compassion is the greatest, scariest and hardest gift you will ever give yourself. It has been said that holding a grudge against another person is like drinking poison and expecting the other person to die. Are you poisoning yourself? This powerful shift is the precursor to the next piece...

Honoring yourself and your gifts

You showing up as yourself is the most incredible gift you can share with the world and the people you love. Knowing the dialect of your desire and being vulnerably brave enough to speak your truth. To show up as exquisitely you and truly be seen. To be loved for your imperfections, not in spite of them.

Take the time to nourish your gifts

It is impossible to be switched on all of the time and create and produce products of your desires consistently. When you don't switch off, you do not nourish your true self and your gifts do not shine as brightly as they could.

Own Your Choices

The choice is yours: allowing and surrendering. No matter what you have been conditioned to believe, it is time to step up and acknowledge how beautiful and powerful you truly are. Vibrant. Shining. Strong. You have been given the gift and the ability to experience sensuous pleasure for a reason - to keep you vital and connected; to yourself, those closest to you, and your community.

Sensuality is a full immersion experience of your senses. Sensuality is how you experience pleasure in your environment. It is the taste of fresh tart raspberries that fall off the vine, the intoxicating aroma of a spring lilac in its short window of deliciousness, the crispness of fresh cotton sheets fresh from the clothes line, the crescendo of your favorite aria coming through your speakers, make it all yours.

Sensuality requires surrender. Fear can often get in the way of that surrender. Fear is a sign that you are getting closer to what you want. Stepping back and postponing sensual maturity only serves to dampen the deluge of desire waiting to flood your newly created space. Until you have a clear vision of what you want and have the courage to go for it, no strategies, blueprints and offers are going to help you. It's time to focus and fuel your vitality.

I was born into this world to help other women find their courage and give voice to their most intimate desires and find their own light through the veil of fear and shame. I fully own and admit that I am a passionate person. I love ideas, new concepts, and deliveries. It brings me so much pleasure. I also admit that following through on all my ideas leaves me exhausted and overwhelmed. And my constant undercurrent is a search for clarity.

Once you set up the expectation that pleasure only happens at the perfect moment, when all the tasks for the day are done, when your bank account is overflowing, when your jeans are a size 32. Once you go to the place of being "right", you've lost the moment. Pleasure is immersion in the NOW. It exists in the silent spaces between breaths, between the doings of life. That is when your pleasure emerges. Claim it. Act on your desires. It is fuel for your vitality. You have all the pleasure you want in you now. Seize it. Step into your feminine. Own your pleasure. Revel in your wildness. Embody your Shakti to the core.

The Goal is to feel good. What are you waiting for?

CHAPTER 8
EMBODIMENT

WHEN A WOMAN reconnects her motions and intelligence somatically to her body and her sexuality, she begins her journey back to wholeness and back to Herself. How do you connect to your feminine at a soul-level? What is your process of moving from the 'doing' of life to the 'being?'

Come face-to-face with the essence of your most sensual self.

Can you remember who you were before the world told you who you should be? Are you still her? What is stirring deep inside you, longing for breath, for birth, for creation? It has once tasted freedom, but has been stifled and strangulated by shoulding, people pleasing, what ifs.

Who you should be is constantly fed by the ideas of modern life, where exhaustion is worn proudly like a badge of honour and withered spirits are filled temporarily with trips to Costco and new Louboutins. These material luxuries wear away quickly and your fragile, delicate self is left to seek cover again. We walk, we talk, yet we are asleep to our passions. Surrounded by shiny distractions, but at what cost? Recognizing the incongruence of our choices is the first step to getting unstuck.

It's possible to feel good.

Really good.

It is yours for the taking when you are ready. You have everything you need to shine, to bloom. It's in you right now.

Sometimes we get so caught up in the Doing of life that we forget about the Being. It is in the quiet moments in-between, the being fully present with another that intimacy is created and expanded. It is necessary to be in our bodies and not living in our heads to cultivate true intimacy and embodiment. To do lists, tasks, jobs. Stop what you are doing right now, take a breath and ask yourself "Am I in a state of being or doing?"

What does it take to move to that place of being, if even for a moment?

You do not have to know how to read the map to begin your journey. Just begin. Your body knows pleasure when it comes across it. How do you begin to connect to sexual energy?

Here are some ways to begin...

1. Immerse your body in water

    Water is a fluid medium, never still. Dynamic. It has an energy all to itself that is essential to life force. Allowing your body to just BE in water and let it move naturally with the tides and ebbs will help you connect to your creative energy. When I am feeling stuck, directionless, stagnant and could binge watch Netflix, I find myself drawn to water. Water is always in flow, when it stagnates it becomes polluted and cannot sustain life. Just like your feminine essence - stagnation breeds stuck-ness, apathy and depression. Find yourself some water and get immersed in its flow. Allow yourself to be. No expectations. Just be. And find your flow.

2. Dance

   Allowing your body to move is a very primal way of connecting to your sensual and creative energy. Ancient rituals of belly dancing were used to prepare women for childbirth; for creation. The rhythmic movements were to support labor, connect to the divine feminine power, your Shakti, and release endorphins. Women connected to their power in the ultimate form of creation. For example, Flamenco, the national dance of Spain, evokes passion, surrender and a primal energy. There is a word to describe this feeling, *duende*, which means to be moved by art on a soulful level. This my sisters, is embodiment; the longing in the singing, the visual dresses, the drums you can feel in your chest, the guitar evoking feelings of intrusion and surrender. This is *duende*. *Duende* is possible for you to feel in your life, every day. This is living below the neck.

3. Orgasm

   Ah, yes. The complete path and connection of sensual and creative energy. Whether alone or with a partner, it is hard to ignore the creative juices that flow once this automatic release has taken place. Our focus becomes clear, we're drunk on feel good hormones and saturated in oxytocin. Ahhh. The Kundalini energy is moving. Unblocked, flowing freely, connecting the dots closed by expectations, by timelines and deadlines. Connection to self, to soulful expression. This is where it comes from.

When you tune into pleasure, you tune into creativity. Into purpose. Your story comes forth naturally. It comes forth with integrity and your raw truth, your uncensored truth emerges. Go ahead. Bathe in creativity. Bathe in passion. See what happens next. The results won't contain themselves to your page. They will permeate your heart and relationships and shields and masks. Let yourself be emotionally naked. Remember that the key is to get in touch with your body.

Multitasking is great everywhere, but the bedroom. A woman must allow herself to bask in her amazing senses taste, touch, smell, sight, and hearing. Not only that, be okay with unabashedly taking sensual pleasure from the sexual experience. Your body is an absolute wonderland that invites you to enjoy sex. It's time you get on board.

Your sexuality is the keystone that supports and nourishes the many roles you play - wife, mother, sister - so you can move closer towards life as a fully integrated person.

Is your default mode strain or ease? Pleasure or obligation?

What is the first thing that runs through your mind when you wake up in the morning?

"I didn't get enough sleep."

"I have so much to do today."

"Gotta check my email."

All these thoughts happen before your feet hit the floor, before life unrolls into your day. It sets the tone for scarcity; not enough time, money, energy, never enough. It becomes a way of being, running to catch up to the endless to-do's of life, work, family, activities. We find ways to do things faster and more efficiently so that we can do more. An endless cycle of chaos.

Often, our heads hit the pillow with the echoes of more scarcity:

"Oh my goodness, I didn't get anything done today."

"I'll just add that to my to-do list tomorrow."

"I am exhausted."

"If only there were more hours in a day."

The wheels never stop spinning. We don't rest. We worry. Insomnia creeps in.

Repeat the same cycle tomorrow.

What is the goal in this? Where does pleasure reside? Is it even on your radar?

Pleasure isn't something we do or get, it's something we are.

It's time for an antidote to scarcity of pleasure.

It's called hedonism; the pursuit of pleasure for the sake of pleasure. But how do you make time for this? Let's disguise it as self-care, a term we are familiar with, but possibly hesitate to practice. Self-care is the time away from life we take to repair our connection with self, to build intimacy in the moments in between breaths. It's about practicing mindfulness and being fully present.

It's about taking 10 seconds in your busy day to make yourself a priority. Like now.

Take 10 seconds and close your eyes, take a deep breath. Exhale deeply. You are a gift to others, to the world to your family: name three ways you are valued or how you have added value to another's experience today. What are three things that are abundant in your life?

Love? Wealth? Health? Time?

Take a second to appreciate them and watch pleasure unfold in your day.

Pleasure can take many forms, sex and orgasm of course. The root of the word sensuality is sense. Pleasure can manifest in the form of sensory awareness, our experience with the environment around us. Think of the intoxicating scent of jasmine, the feel of melting square of divine chocolate in your mouth, the natural sounds that emanate from your body when you taste an exquisite meal. Many of us have been moved to tears by an extraordinarily crafted piece of music written just for us.

That intimate connection, holding the space for pleasure to reveal itself, is the new hedonism, the pursuit of pleasure purely for joy. Can you remember what it was like to be a child, waking up and embracing your day? Before the world censored you and told you how to be, to act? To wake everyday with exquisite joy and embrace each experience without hesitation? The feeling of being all in for the pleasure of the day, to nap on command, exhausted by pure divine exhilaration? And the feeling of resisting bedtime at any cost to take in every second of opportunity for joy and pleasure you could?

So what is it like to be a woman in the world, a woman who knows pleasure who knows how to taste her desires, how to give herself permission to feel those desires to have pleasure in every day? She enjoys sensual moments from the moment she wakes up until the moment she lays head on her pillow at night. How can we create the space to know pleasure and also nurture our families, our relationships, our children, our communities, our workplaces? It can be done. All it takes is a fully embodied YES and the momentum begins.

It's about recognizing that your primary sensual relationship and pleasure begins with you. It's time to nurture that sensual relationship that we have with ourselves and come into full bloom. It is time to create your new pleasure reality. But how do you know which direction to go? Go in the direction of your sensual flow.

It's time to stop flirting and take the plunge, to embrace courage, fear and strength.

To fully dive into life.

Today's reality? It's messy and beautiful. I have touched serenity and happiness with my bare hands. It is exquisite. It's about flexible, but firm boundaries, bravery and trusting intuition. It's about an empathic "No, because my body says so." This is my reality and I am proud that my children and husband embrace my messy, emotional self and love me for it.

How about now?

This very minute this second.

Stop what you're doing and take a breath. Close your eyes.
Fully exhale.
Now open your eyes and consider this question:
what in your environment this very minute inspires desire and feels like pleasure?

Yes, you may be at work, at school, in bed, making supper. What about this very moment brings you pleasure?

Take it all in.
Don't worry. I'll wait...

Did you uncover the pleasure right in front of you? Yes? Fantastic! Soak it up, roll in it, breathe it deep into your lungs and take a mental photograph labeled: feel more of this.

Didn't uncover any beauty, desire or pleasure? Ask yourself a second question: why?

Why are you where you are at this very moment? Is it it of fear, guilt, obligation, necessity? Is your physical environment boxing you in or is your pleasure bounty limited by your thoughts?

Get back to why: what is the script running through your head right now as you search for everyday pleasures?

"I deserve pleasure"

"My desires deserve space"

"I want more of this because it feels right"

Or does it resemble:

"What if I'm caught daydreaming at work?"

"What will they think?"

"This is stupid. I've got deadlines to meet, then I can dabble in my desires, if I have time."

If not now, when? When is an ideal time to inspire a life of met desires, of pleasure for the sake of feeeeelllllling goooooood. Because feeling good if the goal - here, now, today - not later, next week, or when I am successful.

Today is what we have to feel good. Often times we multitask and free up time, only to create new to-do lists and projects when all we really need is breathing room. This room lets us uncover the pleasure that lays before us.

Let's revisit the question:
what about this very moment brings you pleasure?

"The way the sun filters through the glass reminds me of my favourite book."

"The smell of my clothesline dried sheets reminds me of a warm summer hug."

"When I look in the mirror, I am proud of my curves, my wrinkles and my eyes, which tell a story without speaking a word."

Pleasure is everywhere. It is a gift to be able to see the pleasure, the extraordinary in the everyday. You have the capacity to access that gift - in this very moment. Take a breath and slow down to see the beauty before you and *in* you.

Breath this in. It needs to be said again. It needs to be remembered. It needs to be felt.

Pleasure isn't something we do or get, it's something we are.

Your pleasure and desires have a voice. The world requires your voice. If you have uncovered your truth, what are you waiting for? It takes time to fully comprehend the ripple effects of your choices and understanding. Break off the rust keeping you ensnared in its stillness. Speak up. The world is waiting to hear what you have to say. As a woman of words, your sisters are here to support you in reclaiming your voice. Your sensual story is waiting for permission to emerge. Permission granted.

It's about slowing down and being fully present to experience it. It's about being in your body and getting out of your head. It's about putting down the electronic distractions and reconnecting with your body. Stop the distractions and start being present. For some of us this is a real struggle, as it feels unsafe to us, to be alone with ourselves. Your body has so much wisdom. Once you feel safe and trust the inherent wisdom in your body, being fully present, amazing things happen. It's time to break up with external validation and approval. It's time to dump others definition of your success. Embodiment being fully present in your body - the immediate sensory experience of knowing and trusting yourself in the now is the keystone to moving forward to your most awakened self.

Stop falling into patterns of anxiety when opportunities for freedom arise. Restore and explore your relationship with your instincts. The gap between your current reality and the life of your desires seems to be growing more and more every day. But it doesn't have to be. Be brave, dive in and examine and process, the stuff you've buried for so long. Make your desire to wake up bigger than your desire to stay unconscious. Choosing awareness is scary yet necessary. Choosing awareness is embracing sensual flow. It is about deeply integrated pleasure into every moment. It is about diving deep and dropping the stories that no longer work and discovering the freedom that comes with expressing your true feminine desires. Don't allow the *how* to stop you. Trust the process.

This is the time when your whole world turns upside down. Once you've made it through, you're reborn, you're completely rebuilt and everything that you have believed in, everything that you believed you were is not valid anymore. When what is within us comes out, everything changes. It is inevitable. Often what stands in the way is guilt, fear and shame. This ugly trio paralyzes your efforts to get in contact with your sexual and sensual confidence.

Confidence brings clarity and naming your desires is the catalyst. But often, we can't do it alone. Because this awakening is a process, it is a peeling back of layers that requires time and ever-deepening awareness, and in order to keep going deeper, to keep embodying your truth, you need to seek out love and support to hold your hand along the path.

Energy. It is what fuels us. Feminine energy is centripetal energy which spirals up from earth. It draws people in. It is irresistible energy. It's energy coming up from earth and spiraling through our uterus, breasts and hearts and attracting those around us.

Our energy body is comprised of seven chakras, where energy

transforms from emotional to physical body. Each one associated with an organ system and emotional state. It makes us aware of our Somatic wounds. We have a mind body connection so we can heal those somatic wounds. Your Feminine energy is centered in the 2nd chakra, also known as Swadhisthana. It is physically and literally a creative space, with the organs of reproduction and the uterus being in the chakra space. It is the seat of your sensual energy as well as your creativity and femininity.

Creativity is the cousin of sensual energy. This is your creative space. Early programming has us habitually falling into roles and carrying these roles out accordingly. We are programmed to tend to the needs of those relationships we are in. We often become controlled by the fears of the second chakra, like abandonment, financial, status, and family. It gives us our basic survival instincts and intuitions, as well as a desire to create. It houses the habits that keep you small. Creativity is the opposite of stagnation. When we break the stagnation mold and create, our world has personal meaning. Creativity can give us momentum along paths we would have never anticipated and enhance the positive changes happening to carry an idea, onto the next stage of life.

Creativity needs to be used consciously. The second chakra contains the desire and the ability to create life, and a portal for sexual expression. Spiritual connection. Being sensual is being in the moment, in your body, present - a key tenet of embodiment and meditation.

Let's dive in deeper.

What influences and motivates you to make the choices you do, in life, in relationships, in love?

How do you manage your creative energies?

Meditation

Kundalini energy rises in most women about age 40. Its coiled energy sits at the base of the spine, and as it rises, and uncoils, activates the chakras through which it passes. Any unfinished business in each chakra will make itself known during the climacteric period. Carolyn Myss poses that "for women that have had limited sexual pleasure, the blocked Kundalini energy or unused sexual juice may manifest as hot flashes. Unused creative energy or creative conflicts may also be expressed at hot flashes. In women younger than 40, menstrual problems are classic indications that she is in some kind of conflict with being a woman, perhaps believing that her messages about sexuality are confusing and her choices are controlled by others. For instance, a woman may feel sexual desire but feel guilty about it or be unable to speak about it. She may not even be conscious of her inner conflict."

Kundalini energy is managed through yoga and consciousness work. As an alternative to orgasmic release, Kundalini teaches that spiritual ecstasy can be reached through disciplining one's sexual energy, culminating in a spiritual union with the divine. Energetically, orgasm is the release of emotional debris. When there is no release, energy backs up in the systems and without conscious release, can interfere with normal balance.

What does that mean for you recognizing your kundalini energy and how can you cultivate it? It expands awareness, opens into divine states of consciousness, opens your heart space. Tantra is the energy of intimate connection, welcoming and opening to being at one with what is. It may be instinctive, but if we don't nurture it or give it any value, it goes back into hiding.

Get still. Ask yourself what you desire. Listen for the answer.

Your uterus is a literal creative space. You can create babies, books, manifestos, art, businesses. Free up this space. Don't clutter it up with others obligations and fears. This can become a massive overfilled storage closet of shame.

As I have mentioned before, shame is a result of social programming that tells you that you are not enough. It disconnects you from others and tells you that you are inferior. It can have roots in family, in trauma - emotional and physical, in sexual assault, you name it. The second chakra is the storage container for shame. When a woman internalizes and has false ownership of sexuality, physical symptoms show up as external manifestations of internal chaos, of ignoring this innate feminine wisdom.

Let healing work its way through you gently, on its own timeline. Respect this timeline. What unconscious baggage do you store in your body on behalf of others or projected from others? What unresolved relationship issues are taking up space that could be used to nurture your creativity and sensuality?

The sacral chakra is quite literally the cup of life right from where one can create life all the way to the center to where all of one's creative energy is birthed. Sensual energy fuels our creative flow, pleasure, love and wisdom. Your power comes from forging a strong connection with your inner strength and heeding what it wants to say. The element of the sacral chakra is water. It's connection to nature is through flowing water, moonlight and moon bathing. It is strongly tied to our emotions around intimacy and desire. Your movement - however it may manifest itself - is self-care, nourishing, nurturing. When you nourish your creative soul, you become one step closer to what you are looking for. Time is never wasted in the pursuit of your soul's calling.

The awakened woman has too much Divine feminine energy flowing through her to sit still. You have to wake it up. You have to surrender to it.

Chapter 9
Sisterhood and Support

*"I think of writing simply in terms of pleasure. It's the most
important thing in my life, making things. Much as I love
my husband and my children, I love them only because I am
the person who makes these things. I, who I am, is the person
that has the project of making a thing. Well, that's putting
it pompously – but constructing. I do see it in sort of three-
dimensional structures. And because that person does that all
the time, that person is able to love all these people."*

Dame AS Byatt

THE WORLD IS in desperate need for women to experience true sisterhood – loving, deep, nourishing, healing,
supportive. And I know that it's time to heal the wounds
of separation – comparison, jealousy, judgement – among women.

Who gets to see the real you? How do you decide who is safe to
bare your soft, vulnerable underbelly to? Who has earned the right
to hear your desires and fears? As I mentioned earlier, vulnerability
is key to freedom, but it is a privilege for others to hear your story.
Not everyone has earned the privilege. So, how do you decide who
has earned the right to be in your sisterhood?

Instead of seeking solutions, women spend time wondering

why their own needs are not being met. Initiate and follow through on your desires, allows you to enhance your sexual confidence and make bold choices in service to your sexual self.

Who are you? Who do you want to be? Be THAT. Step into it. And go out and do that in every moment. It's time. Your time. Don't delay the party until after the to-do list is done. Time to tap into your true sense of intuition, regain the sacred and create communities of support, all while rewriting and re-imagining how you walk in the world as a sensual woman.

None of your growth, potential and ecstasy is possible to maintain without support. Sisterhood brings support, integration, play, clarity, and healing. It creates a space for healing, time and an opportunity for you to be witnessed in your beauty, your vulnerability and your grief.

An awakened woman knows and owns her sensuality as sacred and loves her own fire. Her fire heats, nourishes and warms others. Her heat heals, supports and refines intuition, creativity and passion. A woman's fire heals. Through this compassionate and personal process, you will change unhealthy emotional patterns and sexual difficulties that have been unconsciously affecting your life, thus revealing your authentic self to create the sex and intimate connection that is right for you. Sexy begins within, let some of that sensuality ooze out onto your skin. Pleasure-seeking women yearning to reconnect with nature and inspired to awaken their inner goddess will be attracted to your energy and power.

You need sexual guides for your sexual life, just like you need doctors for your physical health and mechanics for your car. If you are never willing to invest in your sexual life financially, energetically and with your time, it will stay relatively the same. You will not rise above the sexual mediocrity that most of the masses tell themselves is normal. Yet you can have an extraordinary sexual life. So much is possible and most people never allow themselves to have that because their egos are too big or too sensitive to ask for help or, God forbid, get caught educating themselves about sex.

There was a time that playing and staying small was essential for your survival. It is a survival skill that you may carry with you still. Do you still need to play small in the world and hide your true light? Or can you dump this idea? Tell the truth in every situation and learn to feel how the truth shows up in your body. The truth is where your desires and creation merge. Examine how the truth feels in your body. Is it loud and boisterous, chatty? Or quiet and still, confident? Pleasure is what fuels your body to create and regenerate. It fuels who and what a woman is in all of her brilliance and darkness. Living your passion is the creative force that makes things happen. Stand inside your truth and feel its core sensual fire. Sensuality is the connective tissue that connects you to the universe and others. Your emerging feminine is not logical, in fact it is quite the opposite, intuitive and popping like popcorn as enlightenment makes connection with the now. Trust your inner guidance and don't worry about getting it right. Fearlessly confront whatever stands in the way of your awakening. This is an essential role of belonging to the sisterhood.

Where do we learn about sex/sensuality/intimacy? There are so many positive role models and mentors in our lives and the Sensual Sisterhood brings them together. Whether Maiden, Mother & Crone, we are all experts on our own bodies and experiences. There is so much wisdom to share with one another and The Sensual Sisterhood is the catalyst for expanding discussions, connections and support among women. We meet in person, online, in women's golf circles as well as weekend destination retreats to come together, support one another and provide a sacred space for healing. There is no spiritual affiliation associated with the Sisterhood, only what you bring with you.

I am so excited to share and expand the Sisterhood with you, there is so much that will be revealed through the women who willingly share with each other their struggles and life experiences and courageously create a different reality for themselves. Women show up with an intention to create friendship and connection in their lives. It's about connecting your outer world with your inner vision. Women who bear witness to others' emergence, to sort through all the aspects of their lives and choose what will expand and flourish, and what can be released. Women's friendships are a renewable source of power.

My first experience in a women's sensual circle was a true immersion. I dove in headfirst. I stood in front of a floor length mirror while two women undressed me. It was day 2 of a 3 day retreat with 12 women on the journey back to knowing themselves as sensual beings. 2 days prior, I was on a small ferry taking me to the beautiful gulf island near my home where I was to uncover and return to my true self. I looked on the dock as my husband, a preschooler and an infant waved goodbye and they grew smaller as the boat sailed away. My heart ached, knowing I would miss them and yet also conflicted with the excitement of knowing I would be a new woman upon my return. I felt slightly jealous and nervous too, that they could survive without me, that I was somehow not needed. What I did not recognize at this time was the gift of support that was there for me from my husband, recognizing that I needed the space to know myself as not just a wife and mother, but as a woman. I am blessed that he could see what I could not.

I was picked up at the ferry by the lovely group facilitator who took me to a private residence where we would be spending the weekend. It was a west coast style home, with massive windows on a cliff overlooking the pacific ocean in all its sparking wild green beauty. Little did I know this would be a reflection of my soul in days to come. The other women trickled in slowly over the next few hours, bringing food, blankets and prized possessions to add to the circle. Once we were all settled in, the energy in my belly began to rise, and I knew I would walk out of here a changed woman. As we descended into emotional intimacy and trust with each other, a safe space was created quickly. I was the the youngest of the group at 35, the other ladies ranged from 40-70, and their collective wisdom and confidence was awe inspiring. They had what I wanted: confidence, self-assuredness, a knowing that is beyond words. I wanted a taste. By the end of day one, we had set up our expectations and intentions and created a safe space for expansion. Bring on day 2 and the mirrors.

After a delicious breakfast in the sun, we gathered to do the mirror work. I was simultaneously nauseated and excited at the thought of being naked. With mirrors. With other people present. We broke out into groups of three and started our process. Suppressing dry heaves, I graciously allowed the others to go first. It was a beautiful and moving experience, witnessing others unfolding into self love. They started to melt away their body loathing and replace it with exquisite self love and appreciation. My turn finally arrived and after seeing that the sky did not fall in, I decided to create the space for myself. I must have stared in the mirror for 10 minutes to steady myself before I asked them to take off my shirt for me. It was scary, yes, but also welcoming. They were gentle and supportive and quiet, emanating only love and support for me on this inner journey. I took a deep breath and asked them to remove the rest. Being witnessed in my vulnerability was profoundly moving. I felt seen, I felt empowered, lit up and free. Those two beautiful women were so gracious and welcoming and there was not a single ounce of judgement in the air. Their only job was to create a space for me and write in my journal what I said during the process. In reflection, the transcriptions read: "This is not as bad as I thought. I can do this. I love my eyes, they can see love. I love my full breasts, I can see the blood vessels stand out on them as they nourish my son. I have more hips than I want, and they all allow me to move to dance and express my sensuality through them. They sway when I walk and my feminine speaks for itself. I really like my body, maybe I require

a larger vessel for my work in the world." And just like that I created space for more confidence, self-assuredness and feminine wisdom to surface. And it did. In that moment, surrounded my pure
love, sisterhood and safety. It had always been there. I was just out
of practice. And I have not let go since. It fuels me.

We can spend so much time and energy fighting what we see
- procrastinating, denying ourselves - your sisters will be observers
and show you your blind spots and help you get out of your own
way. They will celebrate what makes you you. You are responsible for
what you see. You get to choose your perspective. Surround yourself
with like-minded women who support your authenticity and cultivate leadership, community and share wisdom.

This sacred sorority offers a space to reclaim connection to your
inner wisdom and get back in touch with your desires. Space to
expand into yourself and cultivate relationships with other women
on the same journey. A healing space to finally exhale and fall into
your truth: nourished, supported, safe. You.

It is a movement of women reclaiming desire, embodying the
truth of who they are and owning their strong, sacred sensual nature.

Chapter 10
Your Journey Home

YOU HAVE MADE your pleasure a priority and fueled every room in your life with your femininity, your power and your innate wisdom. The woman who opened this book at page 1 was all too familiar with shame, guilt, perfectionism and self doubt. Yet you still housed Her, your unique feminine essence, who knows without a doubt that you are capable and loved and able. You are enough as you are, whether you're on page 1 or 101; who you are when you started this book was enough. Enough to make your desires a reality, enough to make room for them to show up, enough to stand up to your old useless beliefs and enough to stand confidently as she is, imperfect and exquisite.

Your vulnerability is your ticket to freedom and accessing your sensuality is the portal to begin your journey. Once you access the portal there is no going back. Only expansion happens from this point forward. What have you given yourself permission to do, be and say in the last 100 pages? What has your YES yielded you? Joy, love acceptance and connection? Keep that shit up. There is no limit to these things. They are abundance. Your joy and connection do not know scarcity. That is only a belief you may have applied to them.

What is the best way to make sure you keep your mama mojo flowing? Stay open and connected with other women. Regularly.

Attend a circle in your community or online. Can't see any? Start one yourself. You will attract exactly the women you need in your life. You are a gift to each other. In each of our lives the maiden, mothers and crones are there for reflecting different levels of experience and wisdom in different domains of our lives and to guide us in our return to Her. No matter what you are experiencing, another woman in your life has experienced that exact same thing. Really. Tap into her knowledge and expertise and tools that helped her navigate her journey back to herself, whether it be her health, relationships, spirituality, child rearing or her professional life. She's been there and can help you navigate your journey back to yourself with her wisdom. The same wisdom you have. It's innate, sometimes we just need to learn the language it's speaking. Weave your awakening into action. Return to Her, to that place inside yourself that intuitively knows what to do and say and feel. That place of pure acceptance and creativity.

The same woman that picked up this book over 100 pages ago is still you. Something inside of you has shifted. Perhaps a belief, an attitude. Maybe you have created more room for what you truly desire and given yourself permission to OWN your desires. The journey is different for all of us. Yet, in the end, we each come home to ourselves and return to Her.

Remember...

The sensually awakened woman

IS awake and alive. She is in awe and has awareness of the immense power that burns within her.

She does not apologize for herself, her power and her sensuality.

She sees through the fog of fear, obligation and guilt that she was handed as part of her cultural inheritance as a woman.

She owns her unlimited possibilities, and all the terrain and flavours of who she is.

She is tuned into her highly responsive body and the depth of her sensations and nuances.

She is unabashedly herself. And proud of it.

Honours the language of her body to make soul centered decisions.

Shows up is her power in a world that tells her to play small.

Her sensuality feels like the ultimate freedom mixed with ease.

The sensually awakened woman accesses her full spectrum of sensual expression.

Feels alive in her skin and her body.

She claims her pleasure and is able to ask for what she needs.

She is ignited and fully alive in every area of her life.

She has been stifled, shamed, defeated and inhibited. Yet stands strong and supported.

She has come face to face with the essence of her most sensual self - and stayed.

She boldly takes up space and delve into the fullness of her femininity.

She owns her deep, wild, erotic womanhood.

She has the perspective to appreciate the joy that already resides within her.

She is fully awakened and alive.

You have risen from slumber, my love. Stay awake.

ACKNOWLEDGMENTS

Thank you, thank you, thank you to:

My one true love Kevin for your unwavering support and love

My kids Sophia and Dylan for giving me space to pursue my passion

My parents for instilling in me duende, the love of the arts and creativity

To my muse, thank you for your gifts and your voice, it is the heart of Return to Her

For the brave women who contributed their sensual stories of awakening to this book

My book coach, Rocky Callen for her editing prowess, enthusiasm, unwavering confidence and belief in my work

My friend Kimberly Lin Pollard for our weekly writing dates to keep each other accountable

My cover designer James at goonwrite.com for capturing what it means to Return to Her

Damonza.com for formatting my work

And my sisterhood - Cheri, Kim, Kelsey, Karen, T, Barbara, Shaeah, and all the women in my life in The Sensual Sisterhood. I love you all beyond measure.

ABOUT THE AUTHOR

Lesley Stedmon is inspiring women to turn up the volume of their sensuality. As a writer, speaker, RN and sexual empowerment coach, Lesley supports women in surrendering to their sensual stories and and owning their authentic sensual expression. She is the creator of the Sensually Awakened Woman, creating safe workshop spaces for women to be and know all of themselves. Lesley lives on beautiful Vancouver Island, BC with her awesome husband and kids. Find Lesley's musings and videos at www.lesleystedmon.com

60459125R00068

Made in the USA
Charleston, SC
02 September 2016